MCQs in CARDIOLOGY

MCQs in CARDIOLOGY

David A. Sandler, MD, MRCP
*Lecturer in Medicine, University Hospital,
Queens Medical Centre, Nottingham*

and

Gerald Sandler, MD, FRCP
*Consultant Physician, District General Hospital,
Barnsley, South Yorkshire*

with a Foreword by
Douglas A. Chamberlain, MA, MD, FRCP
*Consultant Cardiologist, Royal Sussex County Hospital,
Brighton*

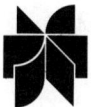

KLUWER ACADEMIC PUBLISHERS
DORDRECHT / BOSTON / LONDON

Distributors

for the United States and Canada: Kluwer Academic Publishers, PO Box 358, Accord Station, Hingham, MA 02018-0358, USA
for all other countries: Kluwer Academic Publishers Group, Distribution Center, PO Box 322, 3300 AH Dordrecht, The Netherlands

ISBN 0-7923-8938-7

Copyright

© 1990 by Kluwer Academic Publishers

All rights reserved. No part of this publication may be reproduced, stored in a retrieval system, or transmitted in any form or by any means, electronic, mechanical, photocopying, recording or otherwise, without prior permission from the publishers, Kluwer Academic Publishers BV, PO Box 17, 3300 AA Dordrecht, The Netherlands.

Published in the United Kingdom by Kluwer Academic Publishers, PO Box 55, Lancaster, UK.

Kluwer Academic Publishers BV incorporates the publishing programmes of D. Reidel, Martinus Nijhoff, Dr W. Junk and MTP Press.

Printed and bound by Butler and Tanner Ltd., Frome and London.

CONTENTS

Foreword   *Douglas A. Chamberlain*   vi

	Question no.	*Answer page no.*
Angioplasty	*1*	34
Aortic dissection	*2–3*	35
Arrhythmia	*4–13*	35
Cardiac surgery	*14–15*	40
Cardiomyopathy	*16–17*	41
Cardiotoxicity	*18*	42
Clinical examination	*19–22*	43
Congenital heart disease	*23–28*	44
Coronary spasm	*29*	48
Driving licence and heart disease	*30–32*	48
ECG	*33–35*	50
Fibrinolysis	*36–39*	51
Heart block	*40–41*	52
Hyperlipidaemia	*42*	53
Hypertension	*43–44*	53
Infective endocarditis	*45–48*	54
Mitral valve prolapse	*49–50*	56
Myocardial infarction	*51–61*	57
Myocarditis	*62–63*	62
Pericarditis	*64–65*	63
Physiology	*66*	64
Resuscitation	*67–68*	65
Rheumatic heart disease	*69–77*	66
Therapeutics	*78–96*	71
MCQs for General Practitioners	*97–110*	80
References		89

FOREWORD

Multiple choice questions can be used equally well to test knowledge or to acquire it. As a method of learning they have several advantages over conventional textbooks. The element of challenge can make it enjoyable; it is efficient because that which is known can be passed over quickly; it is good practice for those who face examinations. Moreover the format is well suited for 'dipping', not a small consideration for those with over busy work schedules.

Cardiology lends itself particularly well to multiple choice questions. We are fortunate that ours is a speciality that is now rich in fact and depends correspondingly little on opinions that can be contentious. This book capitalises on this advantage. A vast amount of information has been packed into sections that are divided conveniently under 25 major topic headings. It matters little that some of the answers provided in the second section seem not to offer a straightforward 'correct' or 'incorrect' judgement that would be appropriate for any formal test of knowledge. They do better, by providing both the relevant facts and useful background information that is well researched and informative.

Sensible multiple choice questions are difficult to write: let those that doubt this fact try their hands! The authors are therefore to be congratulated on producing a particularly useful manual. It is likely to achieve popularity as an effective means of instruction in a rapidly expanding speciality, and is suitable for physicians at all levels, either in general medicine or in cardiology.

Douglas A. Chamberlain

ANGIOPLASTY

1. Percutaneous transluminal coronary angioplasty: (ans. p. 34)

A   is likely to restenose after 3 months
B   is only rarely associated with occlusion during the procedure
C   should be attempted only for single-vessel disease
D   should not be attempted across bypass grafts which have stenosed
E   is a procedure that can be carried out in the X-ray department of most district general hospitals

AORTIC DISSECTION

2. Dissection of the aorta: (ans. p. 35)

A   is frequently associated with hypertension
B   is a congenital abnormality
C   may result from cocaine abuse
D   usually starts with an intimal tear in the descending thoracic aorta
E   is best diagnosed by aortography

3. Dissection of the aorta: (ans. p. 35)

A   has a very high mortality
B   rarely results in cardiac tamponade
C   should be treated with hypotensive medication
D   may be treated conservatively
E   may be complicated by myocardial infarction

ARRHYTHMIA

4. When considering the likely mechanisms or causes of arrhythmias: (ans. p. 35)

A   triggered automaticity is the commonest mechanism for a supraventricular arrhythmia
B   a broad complex tachycardia is most likely to be supraventricular tachycardia with aberrant conduction
C   antegrade flow through the bundle of Kent is the cause of the tachycardia in WPW syndrome
D   sinus tachycardia is unlikely if the ventricular rate is above 100
E   a narrow complex arrhythmia at a rate of about 150/min is likely to be atrial flutter

5. Ventricular tachycardia (see Figure): (ans. p. 36)

A   requires treatment in all circumstances
B   usually requires DC shock
C   is often associated with hypokalaemia
D   may be treated by bretylium tosylate
E   of the 'torsades de pointes' variety is best treated with amiodarone

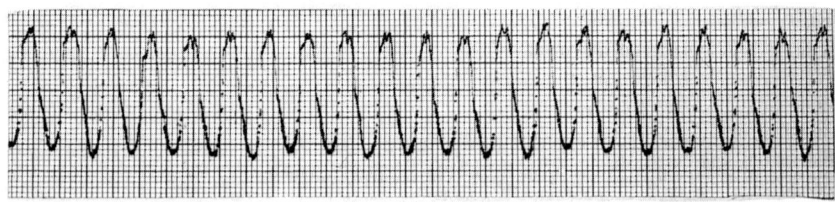

6. In the differentiation between ventricular tachycardia and supraventricular tachycardia with aberrant conduction: (ans. p. 36)

A   the atrial electrogram may help
B   the presence of pre-existing bundle branch block aids differentiation
C   the Rsrl pattern in V1 on the ECG favours a ventricular origin to the tachycardia
D   the deepest QS wave appears in V1–3 in ventricular tachycardia
E   changing wave fronts should lead to a diagnosis of SVT with aberrance

7. When investigating a patient for arrhythmias with a 24 hour ECG recording: (ans. p. 37)

A   any evidence of heart block is abnormal
B   any tachycardia >140/min is significant
C   ventricular bigeminy has no effect on cerebral blood flow
D   asystolic pauses are always significant
E   ventricular ectopic beats are of no importance

8. In the termination of a tachycardia with a pacing wire: (ans. p. 37)

A   underdrive pacing renders a re-entrant circuit refractory
B   overdrive pacing is useful in ventricular arrhythmias
C   the use of an early 'extrastimulus' is a useful method
D   pacing wire should be removed once sinus rhythm is restored
E   ventricular pacing is preferable to atrial pacing most times

9. In attempting to terminate supraventricular tachycardia (see Figure below): (ans. p. 38)

A   ipecachuana may be useful
B   the 'diving reflex' merely requires facial wetting with cold water
C   eyeball pressure is effective
D   carotid sinus massage should be performed with the patient sitting
E   the Valsalva manoeuvre is the most effective non-pharmacological method of terminating an arrhythmia

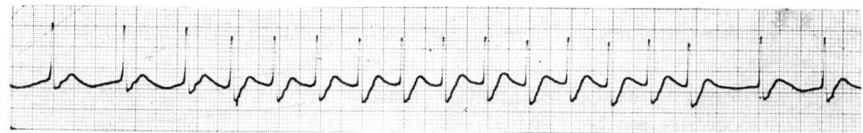

10. In the differentiation of ventricular tachycardia from supraventricular tachycardia with aberrant conduction: (ans. p. 38)

A   a completely regular heart rhythm favours a diagnosis of ventricular tachycardia
B   the presence of p waves favours supraventricular tachycardia
C   atrio-ventricular dissociation confirms ventricular tachycardia
D   vagal stimulation may help in the differentiation by slowing the ventricular rate to allow the p waves to be seen more clearly
E   cannon waves in the neck confirm ventricular tachycardia

11. The Wolff–Parkinson–White syndrome (WPW): (ans. p. 38)

A   atrial fibrillation is caused by atrio-ventricular re-entry
B   a bundle of Kent insertion into the right ventricle gives a predominantly positive ventricular complex in the chest leads
C   may sometimes manifest as a short P–R interval and a normal ventricular complex
D   the Bundle of Kent may insert directly into the ventricular conducting mechanism so accelerating atrio-ventricular conduction
E   associated atrial fibrillation should not be treated with digoxin

12. In the drug treatment of tachycardia: (ans. p. 39)

A   verapamil is effective in converting atrial flutter/fibrillation to sinus rhythm
B   quinidine is effective in preventing supraventricular tachycardia
C   bretylium tosylate is useful in the long-term prevention of ventricular tachycardia
D   atrial flutter is more likely to respond to cardioversion than re-entrant atrial tachycardia
E   verapamil is of no value if the tachycardia is ventricular

13. In atrial fibrillation: (ans. p. 40)

A   hypothyroidism should be considered as a possible cause
B   associated with Wolff–Parkinson–White syndrome digoxin is contraindicated
C   not due to rheumatic heart disease anticoagulation serves no useful purpose
D   cardioversion is the treatment of choice
E   pericarditis may be a likely cause

CARDIAC SURGERY

14. When considering patients with prosthetic valves: (ans. p. 40)

A   tilting disc valves last longer than silastic ball valves
B   warfarin should be prescribed for all mechanical valves
C   tissue valves rarely give rise to structural failure
D   endocarditis is commoner in the mitral position
E   haemolysis is a rare complication

15. Cardiac transplantation: (ans. p. 41)

A   is now rarely complicated by episodes of rejection
B   should not be performed in the presence of pulmonary hypertension
C   should be followed by lifelong immunosuppression
D   is commonly complicated by bacterial infection
E   is not usually followed by atheroma in the donor heart

CARDIOMYOPATHY

16. Sarcoid heart disease: (ans. p. 41)

A   affects the heart valves as well as the myocardium
B   presents most commonly as ventricular arrhythmias
C   should not be treated with steroids because of the likelihood of left ventricular aneurysm developing
D   is best diagnosed by subendocardial biopsy
E   cannot be diagnosed by echocardiography

17. In puerperal cardiomyopathy (PCM): (ans. p. 42)

A   the condition occurs early in the puerperium
B   it usually presents in the first pregnancy
C   toxaemia of pregnancy is a predisposing cause
D   excessive salt intake is often a predisposing factor
E   prednisolone is indicated for treatment

CARDIOTOXICITY

18. Doxorubicin cardiotoxicity: (ans. p. 42)

A can be either acute or chronic
B may be fatal
C is related to the dose of doxorubicin used
D is best monitored by regular measurement of the systolic time intervals, especially the ratio of the pre-ejection period to the left ventricular ejection time
E is less likely if continuous intravenous infusion is used instead of intermittent bolus injections

CLINICAL EXAMINATION

19. When auscultating the first heart sound: (ans. p. 43)

A the tricuspid first sound precedes the mitral sound
B inspiration brings the mitral and tricuspid heart sounds together
C it may sound softer in conditions with a short P–R interval
D it may be widely split in severe mitral stenosis
E will be softened if aortic stenosis is present also

20. When listening to added sounds on auscultation of the heart: (ans. p. 43)

A the third heart sound is due to ventricular filling during atrial systole
B a fourth heart sound is a feature of fast atrial fibrillation
C a gallop rhythm is rare in normal hearts after the neonatal period
D a fourth sound is present in hypertension
E a third sound is of no significance in patients under the age of 30

21. When auscultating the second heart sound: (ans. p. 43)

A pulmonary valve closure precedes aortic closure
B the two components are widely split in pulmonary stenosis
C the second sound usually appears single in atrial septal defects
D an absent second sound may indicate a patent ductus arteriosus
E it may be palpable in transposition of the great vessels

22. When examining the arterial pulse: (ans. p. 44)

A   a dicrotic pulse may be present in febrile states
B   a small volume, collapsing pulse is not a feature of aortic valve disease
C   a large volume collapsing pulse is diagnostic of aortic regurgitation
D   a rise in pressure on inspiration represents pericardial construction
E   pulsus alternans represents mixed aortic valve disease

CONGENITAL HEART DISEASE

23. In considering the natural history of congenital heart disease: (ans. p. 44)

A   ventricular septal defects rarely require surgical closure
B   the common type of atrial septal defect (ostium secundum) usually closes spontaneously in adult life
C   patent ductus arteriosus in full term infants rarely gives rise to any significant clinical problems
D   coarctation of the aorta is rarely associated with any other congenital cardiac defect
E   patients with Fallot's tetralogy usually have a normal life span

24. In a patient with congenital heart disease: (ans. p. 45)

A   a rise in pulmonary artery blood pressure is usually found if coarctation of the aorta is present
B   increased oxygen saturation of the blood in the right atrium suggests a ventricular septal defect
C   a patent ductus arteriosus raises the oxygen saturation in the pulmonary artery
D   due to Fallot's tetralogy the oxygen saturation in the right ventricle is increased
E   the right ventricular pressure is higher than the left ventricular pressure in Eisenmenger's syndrome associated with a ventricular septal defect

25. Coarctation of the aorta: (ans. p. 46)

A usually presents clinically between the ages of 15 and 30
B is rarely associated with other congenital cardiac lesions
C shows rib notching earliest in the first and second ribs
D may be complicated by cerebrovascular accidents
E has a good foetal prognosis in pregnancy

26. Patent ductus arteriosus (PDA) (see Figure): (ans. p. 47)

A is present in about 50% of premature babies
B rarely occurs as a result of maternal rubella in pregnancy
C often presents as heart failure in the neonatal period
D may eventually lead to Eisenmenger's syndrome
E may be closed by infusion of prostaglandin in the neonatal period

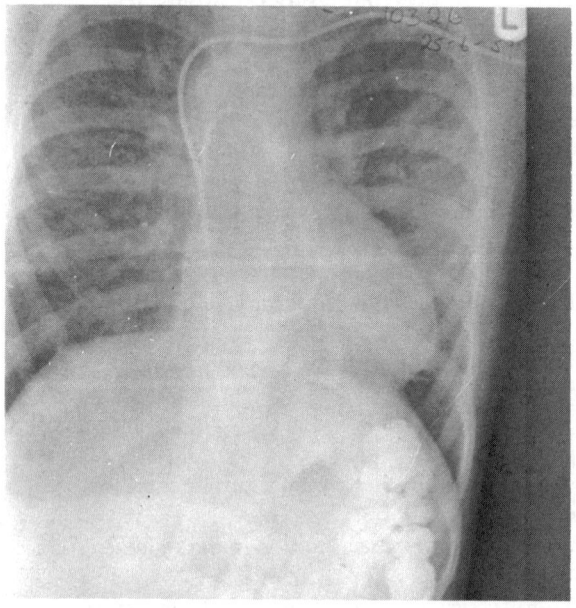

Patent ductus arteriosus – catheter passing through ductus into aorta

27. **In Fallot's tetralogy:** (ans. p. 47)

A   a right-sided aortic arch is common
B   cyanosis is present from birth
C   an increased 'a' wave is seen in the jugular venous pulse
D   the best treatment is a one-stage operative procedure in early life
E   squatting improves the breathlessness

28. **When considering patients with congenital heart disease:** (ans. p. 47)

A   the incidence is about 1 per 1000 live births
B   an atrial septal defect is the most common congenital heart lesion
C   spontaneous closure of a VSD occurs in most patients
D   a VSD results in pulmonary hypertension
E   patent ductus arteriosus and VSD commonly co-exist

CORONARY SPASM

29. **In coronary artery spasm:** (ans. p. 48)

A   there is a resultant tachycardia
B   there is little effect on intraventricular pressure
C   coronary arteriography at rest is usually normal
D   the aetiological factor is an abnormality of smooth muscle in the coronary artery walls
E   myocardial oxygen demand increases before the episode of chest pain

DRIVING LICENCE AND HEART DISEASE

30. A patient with valvular heart disease may not hold a PSV or HGV licence if: (ans. p. 48)

A   the ECG is abnormal
B   medical treatment has been prescribed
C   cardiomegaly is present
D   the patient is not in sinus rhythm
E   operative repair has been necessary

31. The following debar a patient from holding an HGV or PSV licence: (ans. p. 49)

A   paroxysmal atrial flutter/fibrillation
B   sustained atrial flutter/fibrillation
C   supraventricular tachycardia
D   hypertension
E   permanent pacemaker for complete heart block

32. A person may not hold a PSV or HGV licence if: (ans. p. 49)

A   an exercise test is positive
B   an ECG shows Q waves
C   the ECG is normal following a previous infarction
D   there is peripheral vascular disease
E   there is cardiomegaly on a chest X-ray

ECG

33. When studying the ECG: (ans. p. 50)

A   a cardiac axis of >-30 degrees represents left axis deviation
B   left axis deviation is not associated with a secundum ASD
C   right axis deviation commonly co-exists with an ostium primum atrial septal defect
D   left axis deviation is a sign of block in the posterior hemi-bundle
E   pulmonary stenosis may cause left axis deviation

34. With regard to the QT interval on an ECG: (ans. p. 50)

A   it normally becomes shorter with exercise
B   it is normally < 0.42 seconds
C   the Romano–Ward syndrome is recessively inherited
D   the hereditary syndromes of prolongation are responsible for sudden death in young adults
E   hereditary prolongation can be controlled only with the implantation of a permanent pacemaker

35. In the prolonged QT syndrome: (ans. p. 50)

A   exercise shortens the QT interval
B   the duration of the QT interval will depend on the heart rate
C   there may be associated deafness as in the Romano-Ward syndrome
D   associated with ventricular tachycardia β-blockers should be avoided as they cause further prolongation of the QT interval and perpetuate the arrhythmia
E   further prolongation of the QT interval can be caused by hyperkalaemia and hypercalcaemia

FIBRINOLYSIS

36. Myocardial infarction: For the major trials of fibrinolytic therapy in acute myocardial infarction listed below, all of which showed a reduction in mortality in treated patients compared to controls, attempt to match the therapy used and the time after symptom onset that allowed patient inclusion. (ans. p. 51)

A   GISSI   *Lancet*, 1987, 1:392
B   ISAM   *N. Engl. J. Med.*, 1986, 314:1465-71
C   ISIS 2   *Lancet*, 1988, 2:349-60
D   AIMS   *Lancet*, 1988, 1:545-9
E   ASSET   *Lancet*, 1988, 2:525-30

Fibrinolytic Drug
(a) Streptokinase
(b) Tissue plasminogen activator
(c) Anisolylated streptokinase-plasminogen complex

Time to Inclusion
(i)   < 5 h
(ii) < 6 h
(iii) < 12 h
(iv) < 24 h

37. With regard to heparin therapy after fibrinolytic administration: (ans. p. 51)

A heparin should always be used after fibrinolytics
B heparin does not reduce platelet activation
C heparin reduces the incidence of rethrombosis
D heparin induces platelet thrombosis
E heparin inhibits fibrin formation on platelet surfaces

38. The ASSET study[1] (Anglo-Scandinavian Study of Early Thrombolysis): (ans. p. 52)

A compared tissue plasminogen activator (TPA) to streptokinase in acute myocardial infarction
B involved the use of anticoagulation post-thrombolysis
C showed a reduction in mortality after fibrinolysis
D showed that patients without ECG changes at entry had a reduced mortality
E showed an increased incidence of stroke in those given TPA

39. The fibrinolytic pathway is illustrated in the Figure below. Please indicate where in the pathway the items named on the next page appear:

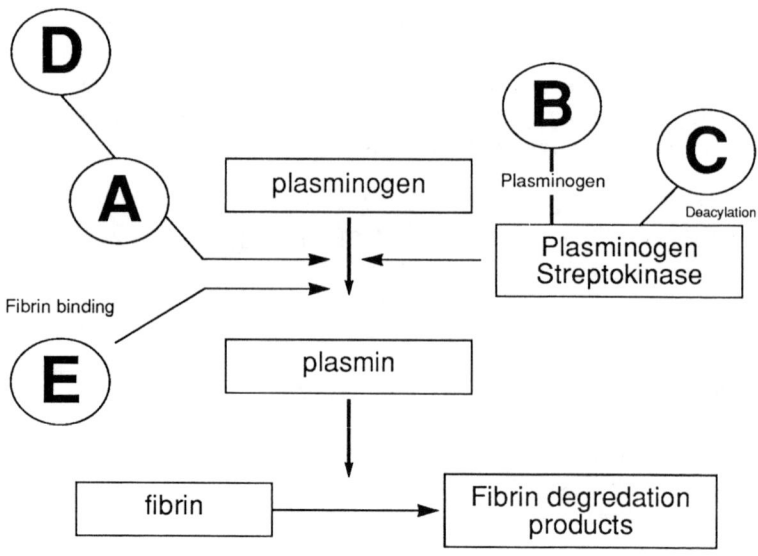

A streptokinase
B APSAC (anisolylated plasminogen–streptokinase activator complex)
C urokinase
D TPA (tissue plasminogen activator)
E prourokinase

HEART BLOCK

40. Left bundle branch block: (ans. p. 52)

A may be associated with an exaggerated 'q' wave in the left precordial leads
B is of no prognostic significance
C may be diagnosed by left axis deviation alone in the ECG
D may sometimes cause right axis deviation in the ECG
E is common in atrial or ventricular septal defects

41. A Stokes–Adams attack (see Figure): (ans. p. 53)

A is often preceded by an aura
B may precipitate a grand mal convulsion
C is associated with pallor
D is followed by a rapid return to normal consciousness once the circulation is restored
E may result in prolonged unconsciousness

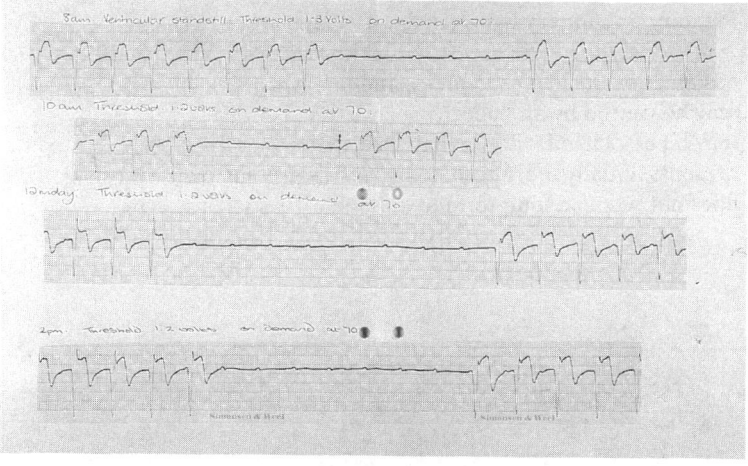

HYPERLIPIDAEMIA

42. In the treatment of hyperlipidaemia: (ans. p. 53)

A nicotinic acid acts by binding bile acids in the bowel
B fibrates are more effective than nicotinic acid in reducing cholesterol levels
C cholestyramine reduces the absorption of digoxin
D gemfibrozil may inhibit the action of warfarin
E clofibrate may increase the incidence of carcinoma especially affecting the bowel

HYPERTENSION

43. Conn's syndrome: (ans. p. 53)

A occurs equally in males and females
B presents most often to the doctor with symptoms of hypokalaemia
C is usually associated with a normal random serum potassium level unless salt-loading is carried out
D associated with an adrenal adenoma can be differentiated from bilateral adrenal hyperplasia by postural studies
E treated surgically by removal of the adenoma will result in normal or greatly improved blood pressure in about 75% of patients

44. Primary pulmonary hypertension (PPH): (ans. p. 54)

A has an equal incidence in males and females
B may be caused by an underlying collagen disorder
C may be associated with Raynaud's disease
D presents initially more commonly with symptoms than with signs
E does not respond long-term to pulmonary vasodilator drugs

INFECTIVE ENDOCARDITIS

45. Infective endocarditis: (ans. p. 54)

A   rarely affects a previously normal heart valve
B   *Streptococcus viridans* is the putative infecting agent in most cases
C   multiple infection is seen only in drug addicts
D   should initially be treated with two antibiotics
E   should be treated for 6 weeks

46. In which of the situations mentioned below should the numbered recommendations be made as prophylaxis against endocarditis in patients with valvular disease: (ans. p. 55)

A   dental extraction under general anaesthetic in a patient allergic to penicillin
B   a patient undergoing bronchoscopy with no drug allergy
C   a patient about to have genitourinary surgery under general anaesthetic
D   a patient with a penicillin allergy about to undergo upper GI endoscopy
E   a patient having an obstetric procedure

Antibiotic regimes
(i)   amoxycillin 3 g orally, 1 hour before procedure
(ii) amoxycillin 1 g i.m. before induction and 500 mg orally 6 hours later
(iii) lincomycin 600 mg 1 hour before induction and 6 hours later
(iv) vancomycin 1 g i.v. over 1 hour then gentamicin 120 mg i.v. just before induction
(v)   amoxycillin 1 g i.m. and gentamicin 120 mg i.m. just before and amoxycillin 500 mg 6 hours later.

47. Libman–Sacks endocarditis: (ans. p. 55)

A   is a common complication of systemic lupus erythematosus
B   almost always affects the mitral valve only
C   manifests histological lesions which are identical with those of marantic endocarditis
D   may lead to the development of mitral stenosis long-term
E   never leads to infective endocarditis

48. Infective endocarditis: (ans. p. 56)

A   may occur in congenital heart disease and atrial septal defect is then the commonest defect likely to be involved
B   is associated with a positive blood culture in only 20%
C   is sometimes a complication of malignant disease
D   is now caused more frequently by staphylococci than by *Streptococcus viridans*
E   should be treated surgically if fungal endocarditis is present

MITRAL VALVE PROLAPSE

49. The floppy mitral valve syndrome (mitral valve prolapse): (ans. p. 56)

A   occurs in less than 1% of the normal, asymptomatic population
B   involves both leaflets of the valve and the chordae
C   exhibits an impulse suggesting a double apex beat
D   is responsible for the mid-systolic click that is present on auscultation
E   the murmur becomes softer after amyl nitrite, which distinguishes it from hypertrophic obstructive cardiomyopathy, which has a similar murmur

50. Mitral valve prolapse: (ans. p. 57)

A   occurs in up to 20% of the population
B   may produce a third heart sound in diastole resembling the opening snap of mitral stenosis
C   is usually benign and does not affect prognosis
D   is due to a localised abnormality of the mitral valve
E   may be associated with mitral regurgitation especially after myocardial infarction

MYOCARDIAL INFARCTION

51. In the ISIS 1 trial (first international study of infarct survival)[2]: (ans. p. 57)

A   atenolol was compared to aspirin in acute myocardial infarction
B   atenolol was given as an oral agent for 1 month
C   patients were enrolled up to 6 hours after onset of symptoms
D   atenolol reduced the incidence of ventricular fibrillation
E   atenolol reduced mortality

52. The ISIS 2 study (second international study of infarct survival)[3]: (ans. p. 57)

A   compared streptokinase (SK) with aspirin in acute myocardial infarction
B   recruited patients up to 6 hours from onset of major symptoms
C   showed no reduction of mortality in those given aspirin alone
D   showed synergy in effect on mortality with combined therapy
E   showed a reduced mortality only in patients younger than 70

53. The ST segment depression seen in the ECG leads other than those subtending the area of acute myocardial infarction: (ans. p. 58)

A   is an electrical phenomenon
B   does not reflect the size of the infarction
C   identifies coronary artery disease in other sites
D   identifies patients at higher risk
E   is related to findings on exercise testing

54. Pericardial effusion after a myocardial infarction: (ans. p. 58)

A   is a frequent complication
B   is associated with an increased mortality
C   tends to resolve rapidly without treatment
D   is indicated by a posterior echo-free space on echocardiography
E   is related to the healing that follows the infarction

55. Right ventricular infarction: (ans. p. 59)

A   is an uncommon pathological finding at autopsy
B   is diagnosed on the ECG by ST elevation in lead V1
C   may frequently result in cardiogenic shock
D   associated with cardiac failure may not improve on diuretics
E   has clinical findings similar to those of left ventricular failure

56. In acute myocardial infarction: (ans. p. 59)

A   thrombotic occlusion follows plaque rupture
B   the initiating event is haemorrhage into the plaque
C   total occlusion of the infarct-related artery always results in transmural infarction
D   thrombolytic therapy increases the arterial lumen
E   injury deep in the arterial wall may be the mechanism which induces thrombosis

57. In trials of β-blockers after acute myocardial infarction: (ans. p. 60)

A   effects are mediated through their antiarrhythmic potential
B   timolol is of proven value
C   propranolol is of little value
D   early administration of atenolol reduces early death
E   treatment should be continued indefinitely

58. Ventricular septal defect after myocardial infarction: (ans. p. 60)

A   usually affects the anterior or apical segment of the septum
B   usually involves the mitral valve
C   is often followed by a septal aneurysm
D   usually occurs after the first 3 days
E   is not usually associated with a significant increase in mortality

MCQs in CARDIOLOGY

59. Q wave and non-Q wave infarction: (ans. p. 61)

A the presence of a Q wave always indicates a transmural myocardial infarction
B non-Q wave infarction is more common in the younger patients
C the prognosis is better in non-Q wave infarction than if a Q wave is present
D Q wave infarction is more common than non-Q wave
E diltiazem improves the prognosis of the infarction providing it is non-Q wave

60. Subendocardial myocardial infarction: (ans. p. 61)

A leaves the QRS complexes on the ECG unchanged
B may be followed by a transmural infection
C is related to coronary vascular resistance
D may be caused by valvular heart disease
E may follow successful resuscitation from cardiac arrest

61. In myocardial infarction with normal coronary arteries: (ans. p. 62)

A there is usually a history of previous angina
B the majority of patients are non-smokers
C the prognosis is better than in myocardial infarction due to coronary atherosclerosis
D coronary spasm is the most likely cause
E most patients will show a positive post-infarction exercise tolerance test

MYOCARDITIS

62. In patients with myocarditis: (ans. p. 62)

A a viral aetiology is usual
B general viral infections are rarely associated with cardiac involvement
C males are affected more than females
D the ECG is diagnostic
E treatment with immunosuppressives should be given early

63. In cardiac involvement with neurological disorders: (ans. p. 62)

A   Duchenne's muscular dystrophy is usually associated with disorders of atrio-ventricular conduction
B   atrial tachyarrhythmias are the usual problem in facio-scapulo-humeral muscular dystrophy (Landouzy–Déjèrine)
C   the myocardium is rarely involved in myotonia dystrophica (Steinert's disease)
D   in myotonia congenita (Thompsen's disease) the heart is often affected and is the usual cause of death
E   in Friedreich's ataxia malignant ventricular arrhythmias commonly occur due to associated hypertrophic cardiomyopathy which is a feature of the condition

PERICARDITIS

64. Chronic constructive pericarditis: (ans. p. 63)

A   is usually caused by tuberculous infection
B   is diagnosed primarily by a prominent 'x' descent in the jugular venous pulse in the absence of a corresponding 'y' descent
C   is often associated with a pulsus paradoxus
D   can be differentiated from restrictive cardiomyopathy (e.g. amyloid, endomyocardial fibrosis) by the presence of left ventricular as well as right ventricular dysfunction
E   has a better prognosis with surgical than medical treatment.

65. In pericarditis: (ans. p. 64)

A   the heart size may be reduced on chest X-ray
B   if a paradoxical pulse occurs it suggests co-existent heart failure
C   a possible cause may be hydralazine
D   bronchial breathing may be heard at the left lung base
E   a fall of the jugular venous pressure on inspiration with absence of the 'x' descent (Kussmaul's sign) indicates cardiac tamponade.

PHYSIOLOGY

66. Atrial natriuretic factor: (ans. p. 64)

A   is mainly secreted in the left atrial appendage
B   production is increased if salt intake is inadequate
C   stimulates plasma renin activity and so leads to an increase of blood pressure
D   is always elevated in the blood in heart failure, irrespective of whether it is left or right sided
E   rises with effective diuretic treatment of heart failure

RESUSCITATION

67. In the recently issued guidelines for cardiopulmonary resuscitation (see *Br. Med. J.*, August 1989): (ans. p. 65)

A   defibrillation plays no part in patients with asystole
B   lignocaine is given immediately after the first DC shock for ventricular fibrillation
C   CPR should be continuous throughout resuscitation
D   the failure of one anti-arrhythmic drug should be rapidly followed by the administration of a further agent
E   medication may be administered through an endotracheal tube

68. Patients who remain unconscious after defibrillation from ventricular fibrillation: (ans. p. 65)

A   should be nursed in a 'head down' position until they regain consciousness
B   should have their blood sugar closely monitored
C   may be improved by hyperventilation
D   should be taken off ventilation as soon as possible
E   may manifest the signs of lignocaine intoxication

RHEUMATIC HEART DISEASE

69. In a patient with aortic valve stenosis: (ans. p. 69)

A   there is often a prominent, negative p wave in V1 of the ECG
B   a calcified valve may be seen in younger patients below the level of the oblique fissure on a chest X-ray
C   the appearance of the valve on M mode echocardiography gives a good assessment of the severity of the stenosis
D   urgent valve replacement is necessary once diagnosis is made
E   of congenital origin, this is usually associated with a ventricular septal defect and/or pulmonary stenosis

70. Mitral stenosis: (ans. p. 69)

A   is never a congenital lesion of the heart
B   most commonly follows an infection with a group C streptococcal organism
C   is best differentiated from an atrial myxoma simulating mitral stenosis by angiocardiography
D   is characterised by fatigue, which may be the presenting symptom
E   may be associated with hoarseness

71. In mitral stenosis: (ans. p. 67)

A   the degree of stenosis of the valve is reflected in the loudness of the first heart sound
B   the position of the opening snap in the cardiac cycle reflects the severity of stenosis
C   more severe stenosis causes shorter diastolic murmurs
D   is never associated with a third heart sound
E   is commonly associated with chronic bronchitis

MCQs in CARDIOLOGY

72. In mitral regurgitation: (ans. p. 67)

A the murmur may be loudest at the left sternal edge
B the murmur is loudest in the back if the posterior chordae have ruptured
C the best view of mitral regurgitation at catheter is in the left anterior oblique position
D the extent of the 'v' wave at cardiac catheter is proportional to the severity of the regurgitation
E has a good prognosis in the presence of good LV function

73. Aortic regurgitation: (ans. p. 67)

A has a good prognosis if medically treated
B may be caused by rupture of a coronary sinus aneurysm
C may be associated with a pulmonary AV fistula
D is rarely associated with a normal ECG appearance
E the chest X-ray may show calcification in the aorta

74. In rheumatoid heart disease: (ans. p. 69)

A pericardial effusion is an uncommon manifestation
B the aortic valve is the one most likely to be affected
C myocarditis is unlikely to occur
D the commonest ECG abnormality is an inverted T wave
E associated coronary artery disease is no more common than in matched controls

75. In aortic regurgitation: (ans. p. 69)

A the Graham-Steel murmur may be confused with the murmur of mitral stenosis
B a pulsus alternans suggests co-existing aortic stenosis
C bobbing of the head (De Musset's sign) may occur
D auscultation of the femoral artery may be helpful in diagnosis
E the typical early diastolic murmur is reduced by squatting and enhanced by the Valsalva manoeuvre

76. Mitral regurgitation: (ans. p. 70)

A may be a manifestation of pseudoxanthoma elasticum
B in Hurler's syndrome is due to elongation and rupture of the chordae tendineae
C in Marfan's syndrome is produced by stretching of the mitral annulus
D in left ventricular failure is caused solely by dilation of the mitral ring
E caused by infiltrative conditions such as amyloid, sarcoid and neoplasm, rarely involves the papillary muscle

77. Aortic stenosis: (ans. p. 70)

A often produces a bisferiens pulse
B is always associated with a reduced or absent second heart sound
C may occur in a congenitally bicuspid valve
D can present as amaurosis fugax
E often causes angina in the absence of associated disease of the coronary arteries

THERAPEUTICS

78. When considering which ACE inhibitor to use: (ans. p. 71)

A enalapril should not be used if liver disease is present
B captopril contains sulphydryl groups which may be responsible for its side-effects
C all are contraindicated in diabetic patients
D enalapril causes proteinuria in congestive cardiac failure and should therefore be avoided
E a skin rash with one ACE inhibitor rules out the use of another

MCQs in CARDIOLOGY

79. When considering whether to use a β-blocker or a calcium blocker in the treatment of hypertension, the decision may be influenced by: (ans. p. 71)

A calcium antagonists are safe in asthmatic patients
B both calcium channel blockers and β-blockers unfavourably alter the lipid profile
C all the calcium blockers aggravate cardiac failure
D nifedipine is relatively safe in digitalis toxicity
E all calcium blockers should be avoided in obstructive cardiomyopathy

80. Nitrates: (ans. p. 72)

A are effective in the treatment of angina associated with hypertrophic obstructive cardiomyopathy
B are contraindicated in constrictive pericarditis
C should be avoided in anterior myocardial infarction
D should not be given to patients with glaucoma
E may be associated with a significant withdrawal syndrome

81. In using a combination of anti-arrhythmic drugs: (ans. p. 73)

A lignocaine and β-blockers may be safely administered together
B quinidine and digoxin should not be prescribed together
C sotalol may be combined with amiodarone
D combinations of Class I agents are potentially dangerous
E quinidine should be avoided in patients on diuretics

82. Digoxin: (ans. p. 73)

A is almost totally absorbed after oral administration
B is lipid insoluble
C is strongly bound to plasma proteins
D is eventually metabolised in the liver before excretion
E may be poorly absorbed in hyperthyroidism

83. In using β-blockers: (ans. p. 73)

A   their antiarrhythmic properties are due to prolongation of the action potential in cardiac cells
B   β-blockers with intrinsic sympathomimetic activity (ISA) interfere with sleep patterns
C   metoprolol is the most cardioselective β-blocker and therefore best for asthmatic patients requiring these agents
D   if β-blockers are essential in patients with airways obstruction, a drug with high ISA is preferable to a cardioselective one
E   combined α- and β-blockade by labetalol is more effective in hypertension than propranolol

84. In using β-blockers in clinical practice: (ans. p. 74)

A   they may aggravate angina
B   they may be usefully combined with calcium antagonists in treating angina
C   they are ideal as first line therapy for elderly patients with hypertension
D   young, black hypertensives are best started on β-blockers
E   atenolol is the preferred β-blocker for hypertension

85. When considering the side-effects of β-blockers: (ans. p. 75)

A   withdrawal from therapy because of side-effects is commoner with atenolol than propranolol
B   heart failure induced by therapy is common in practice
C   β-blockers may cause hypertension
D   pindolol causes less fall in cardiac output than other β-blockers
E   pindolol and propranolol both cause dreams by their lipid-solubility and CNS penetration

86. In using a combination of β-blockers with other medication: (ans. p. 75)

A   β-blockers may be added safely to hypertensive patients on clonidine
B   β-blockers should not be combined with reserpine in the treatment of hypertension
C   cimetidine may potentiate the effects of propranolol
D   β-blockers can usefully be combined with nifedipine in hypertension and angina
E   non-steroidal anti-inflammatory agents (NSAIDs) should be avoided

87. When using cardiac glycosides: (ans. p. 76)

A   ouabain acts rapidly whether administered intravenously or orally
B   digitoxin is advantageous as it has a short half-life
C   lantoside C differs from digoxin only in its side-effect profile
D   intravenous digoxin acts within minutes of administration
E   digoxin has a short half-life and therefore has advantages in flexibility of dosage control

88. Sympathomimetics – Dobutamine: (ans. p. 76)

A   administration must be carried out through a large, central vein
B   has a dopaminergic effect on the heart
C   causes the release of noradrenaline within the circulation
D   has little chronotropic effect at therapeutic doses
E   is a peripheral vasodilator

89. When considering the use of inotropic sympathomimetic medication: (ans. p. 76)

A   noradrenaline causes intense vasoconstriction
B   isoprenaline causes an α-receptor-mediated tachycardia
C   dobutamine causes the release of noradrenaline from the heart
D   dobutamine is a peripheral vasodilator
E   dobutamine stimulates both β-1 and 2 receptors

90. Indicate the correct treatment for each of the numbered scenarios below, based on patients with circulatory collapse: (ans. p. 77)

	Pulmonary Capillary Wedge Pressure (PCWP)	Systemic Blood Pressure	Tissue Perfusion
A	>15	Low	Low
B	>15	Normal	Normal
C	<18	Low	Low
D	<18	Normal	Normal
E	<10	Low	Low

Treatment Options
(i) inotrope alone (e.g. dopamine and/or dobutamine)
(ii) inotrope and vasodilator (dopamine + isosorbide 1 mg/h)
(iii) vasodilator alone (isosorbide and/or nitroprusside)
(iv) volume expansion (colloid or crystalloid solutions)
(v) no treatment

91. When considering the action of antiarrhythmic medications, using the Vaughn-Williams classification: (ans. p. 77)

A class IV agents alter the refractory time of the AV node
B the class III agents act by reducing the His-Purkinje refractory time
C the class II agents act predominantly on the β-1 receptors of the ventricular muscle
D all the class I agents increase the refractory period of the His-Purkinje fibres
E pure class I effect is to inhibit the fast sodium current

92. Precautions necessary when starting treatment with ACE inhibitors include: (ans. p. 77)

A using a small test dose first
B monitor serum potassium level
C an intravenous pyelogram before treatment started
D hospital admission is advisable
E stop all diuretics

93. With regard to vasodilator therapy: (ans. p. 78)

A   isosorbide infusions are potent arterial dilators
B   nitroprusside is predominantly an arterial vasodilator
C   salbutamol infusions may induce hyperkalaemia
D   nitroprusside infusions may cause a metabolic alkalosis if continued beyond 48 hours
E   hydralazine therapy causes venodilation and a fall in venous return

94. With regard to the use of sodium nitroprusside in cardiac failure and cardiogenic shock: (ans. p. 78)

A   a hyperthyroid state may be induced
B   should be administered with a concurrent dose of hydroxycobalamin
C   the infusion is hepatotoxic
D   free cyanide is predominantly plasma protein bound before excretion
E   the metabolite is rapidly excreted through the gut

95. Disopyramide: (ans. p. 95)

A   has anti-arrhythmic properties through its class III action
B   is metabolised mainly in the liver
C   has high bio-availability when given orally
D   is inferior to verapamil in controlling the supraventricular tachycardia associated with the Wolff–Parkinson–White syndrome
E   should be used with caution in hypokalaemia

96. Amiodarone: (ans. p. 96)

A   has no effect on the sympathetic receptors in the heart
B   slows the sinus node rate by 20–30% with chronic oral treatment
C   does not have any negative inotropic effects
D   does not precipitate heart failure when used long-term
E   is completely eliminated from the body in 3 weeks after chronic oral dosage

MCQs FOR GENERAL PRACTITIONERS

97. When using β-blockers for cardiac disease: (ans. p. 80)

A   they should not be used in diabetics
B   they should not be used in patients with Raynaud's phenomenon
C   they may be used if co-existent liver disease
D   they may safely to be given to patients about to undergo surgery
E   they should never be given to severely asthmatic patients

98. In using nitrates: (ans. p. 80)

A   mononitrates offer advantages over dinitrates
B   the nitrate patch offers considerable benefits over oral agents
C   nitrates act in angina by reducing coronary spasm
D   their vasodilatory actions are beneficial in cardiac failure
E   they may be more effective in angina as double-therapy with a β-blocker or calcium antagonist, than triple-therapy with both additional drugs

99. A Stokes–Adams attack: (ans. p. 81)

A   is often preceded by an aura
B   may precipitate a grand mal convulsion
C   is associated with pallor
D   is followed by a rapid return to normal consciousness once the circulation is restored
E   may result in prolonged unconsciousness

100. Match the following manifestations of acute rheumatic fever with the incidence figures given: (ans. p. 81)

A	carditis	(a)	80%
B	arthritis	(b)	50%
C	chorea (St Vitus' dance)	(c)	10%
D	erythema marginatum	(d)	5%
E	long-term valvular heart disease	(e)	30%

101. In children with congenital heart disease: (ans. p. 82)

A   atrial septal defects are usually hereditary
B   the fixed splitting of the second sound in atrial septal defect is due to delayed closure of the aortic valve
C   congenital aortic and pulmonary valve stenosis never occur together
D   finger clubbing can be seen immediately after birth if the congenital heart disease is cyanotic
E   a diastolic murmur is more likely to be heard than a systolic murmur in a ventricular septal defect with Eisenmenger's syndrome (reversal of the interventricular shunt)

102. Digoxin: (ans. p. 83)

A   is a chronotropic drug
B   should not be used to treat heart failure if sinus rhythm is present
C   should be used with caution if the patient is also being treated with carbenoxolone for peptic ulcer
D   is especially effective in treating atrial fibrillation associated with the Wolff–Parkinson–White syndrome
E   always requires an assessment of blood urea level before treatment is commenced in an elderly patient

103. Calcium channel blockers: (ans. p. 83)

A   are negative inotropes
B   reduce the afterload on the left ventricle and so improve heart failure
C   slow the production of impulses in the sino-atrial node leading to brachycardia
D   are of value in treating peripheral vascular disease
E   are all contraindicated in patients with heart block

104. There are a number of eponymous signs in aortic regurgitation – match the signs with the eponyms: (ans. p. 84)

Signs
A   visible capillary pulsation in the fingernail beds
B   visible arterial pulsation in the neck
C   bobbing of the head
D   a 'pistol shot' on auscultation over the femoral artery
E   diastolic murmur following distal compression of the femoral artery

Eponyms
(a)   Duroziez's sign
(b)   Traube's phenomenon
(c)   De Musset's sign
(d)   Corrigan's sign
(e)   Quincke's sign

105. When myocardial infarction occurs in an elderly patient: (ans. p. 84)

A   chest pain is rarely the presenting complaint
B   'silent infarction' is common
C   it is rarely associated with severe dyspnoea in the absence of acute LVF
D   it is not particularly associated with a higher mortality
E   benefits from fibrinolytic therapy are minimal

106. In considering hypertension: (ans. p. 85)

A   one of the major benefits of control is the reduction of fatal myocardial infarction
B   the cause is essential in about 50% of the patients presenting in the surgery
C   an intravenous pyelogram is required in very few patients
D   estimation of urinary catecholamine excretion should be done routinely in young patients because of the likelihood of phaeochromocytoma
E   a renovascular cause is likely if the IVP shows a large discrepancy in the size of the two kidneys (>2 cm).

107. Nitrate preparations in angina: (ans. p. 86)

A   act predominantly by arteriolar dilatation resulting in a reduction in work load of the heart
B   will only dilate the coronary arteries if they are free from atherosclerosis
C   inevitably lead to tolerance if long-term therapy is used
D   are changed from the dinitrate to the mononitrate form in the liver
E   are more effective as a spray compared with the sublingual form in the treatment of an anginal attack

108. Diuretics: (ans. p. 86)

A   may adversely affect the lipid profile
B   should always be prescribed with potassium supplements
C   may lead to impotence
D   all act at the same site in the kidney tubules preventing reabsorption of sodium and water
E   may precipitate muscle weakness, especially in elderly patients

109. Diuretics: (ans. p. 87)

A   all act by increasing the excretion of sodium and water
B   can be direct venodilating agents
C   inhibit the renin–angiotensin system
D   thiazides are more effective in lowering blood pressure than loop diuretics like frusemide
E   may all precipitate gout

110. Post-myocardial infarction prophylaxis. In secondary prevention after myocardial infarction: (ans. p. 88)

A   anticoagulation with warfarin is of proven value
B   aspirin is of proven value
C   dipyridamole is of no proven value
D   antiarrhythmics are of proven value
E   sulphinpyrazone prolongs survival

ANSWERS

ANGIOPLASTY

1.
- A – F Restenosis may occur up to 6 months after the procedure; it is most likely in the first month after the angioplasty.
- B – F Acute occlusion occurs in about 8% of patients undergoing this procedure.
- C – F Although single-vessel disease was the first indication for angioplasty, it can now be attempted for multi-vessel disease and also for more than one occlusion in the same vessel.
- D – F Angioplasty is effective in these circumstances and is the method of choice in such patients.
- E – F This procedure should not be attempted without full cardiac surgical facilities readily available in case of dissection of the coronary artery or acute rupture (<5%): although some hospitals in London do perform PTCA without on-site cardiac surgeons, they are close by in other hospitals.

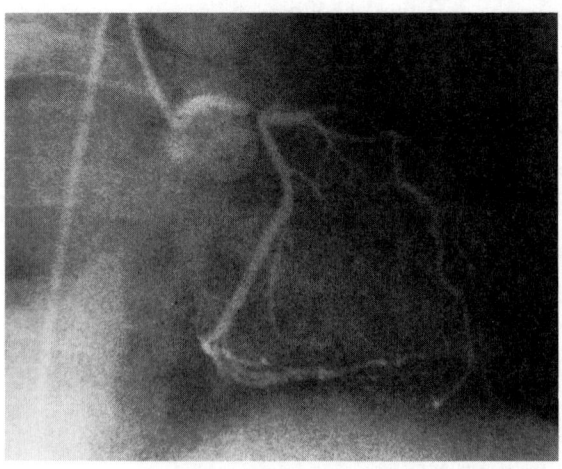

Coronary arteriogram showing stenosis of the left main coronary artery at its bifurcation into the left anterior descending and circumflex arteries. This is the type of lesion ideal for angioplasty.

AORTIC DISSECTION

2.
- **A – T** This is the most common co-existing factor (in 30-45%) and it probably accelerates the normal process of degeneration in the smooth muscle cells of the media and the elastic tissue.
- **B – F** But it is associated with many congenital conditions, particularly those which affect the ascending aorta, e.g. Marfan's, biscuspid aortic valve, coarctation.
- **C – T** Due to the paroxysmal hypertension which occurs with this.
- **D – F** Two-thirds start with an intimal tear in the ascending aorta, possibly becasue of repeated flexion of the aorta during systole, combined with the force of blood being ejected against the intima at the same site.
- **E – F** CT scan, digital subtraction angiogram, magnetic resonance imaging and transoesophageal echo are all likely to supersede aortography, previously regarded as the 'gold standard'.

3.
- **A – F** The mortality is about 30% within the first 2 days.
- **B – F** Dissection with pericardial tamponade is the commonest mode of death in these patients.
- **C – T** The usual target is a systolic pressure of 100 mm or less for the younger patients and 120 mm for the elderly, previously hypertensive patient. This level of pressure can be induced with a labetalol infusion at a rate of 125 μg to 2 mg/minute.
- **D – T** If no complications occur, as is frequent with a posterior dissection. If complications such as loss of pulses, pericardial rupture or aortic regurgitation occur, surgery is a priority.
- **E – T** An ostial stenosis of the right coronary artery may be a complication of a proximal aortic dissection and may itself require treatment.

ARRHYTHMIA

4.
- **A – F** The usual mechanism is a re-entry circuit, either within the AV node or incorporating an accessory pathway.
- **B – F** It is safest to assume that any broad complex tachycardia is ventricular until proven otherwise, especially in any patient with a background of ischaemic heart disease.

    C – F   The supraventricular tachycardia of WPW is caused by the re-entry of an impulse, conducted antegradely through the normal AV node and then retrogradely back up the accessory bundle into the atrium. The less common fast atrial fibrillation sometimes seen with WPW is due to rapid antegrade flow through the bundle of Kent.

    D – F   A regular tachycardia of up to 120 /minute may be a sinus tachycardia but rates higher than this are usually due to SVT.

    E – T   If a patient has a regular tachycardia with a rate of around 140–155, consider atrial flutter with 2:1 block.

5. A – F   Short salvos require no treatment unless causing haemodynamic embarrassment. VT should be treated if at a rate of 120/minute for >30 seconds or >160/minute for 15 seconds.

    B – F   A thump on the chest may work. DC conversion is required if the arrhythmia is rapid (>130) and continuous rather than paroxysmal – and is not the result of digoxin toxicity.

    C – T   And, in patients on long-term diuretics, also with hypomagnesaemia; magnesium sulphate may be included in the treatment regime (10 ml of 50% $MgSO_4$ in 100 ml 5% dextrose given over 60 minutes for every 20 mM potassium infused).

    D – T   This is an option usually reserved for desperate situations: the bretylium tosylate is given as 400 mg in 5% dextrose over 10 minutes – it may however take 20 minutes to be effective and may cause serious hypotension.

    E – F   Drug treament should be avoided as 'torsades de pointes' may be drug-induced. It is best treated by correcting the potassium level, and stopping any drug that may prolong the QT interval (e.g. amiodarone); and also by giving magnesium and sometimes by atrial pacing.

6. A – T   The insertion of a bipolar pacing wire in the high right atrium and the recording of the atrial ECG is of great use, as the 1:1 relationship between P waves and the QRS complex confirms the supraventricular origin of the arrhythmia.

    B – T   If the tachycardia complexes appear similar to the previous appearance of the bundle branch complexes, then the supraventricular origin of the arrhythmia is established.

	C – T	Rsr in V1 is characteristic of ventricular tachycardia, but rSR in V1 is a feature of supraventricular arrythmias.
	D – F	The deepest QS is in V4-5 in ventricular tachycardia. It is in left bundle branch block that the QS is deepest in the septal leads.
	E – F	Changing wave fronts (torsades de pointes) are a characteristic feature of ventricular tachycardia, usually associated with a prolonged QT interval on the ECG.
7.	A – F	First degree block and Wenckebach AV block (in patients with high vagal tone) have been reported in normal individuals.
	B – T	Any heart rates >140/minute or <40/minute are likely to decrease cerebral blood flow and therefore be responsible for symptoms.
	C – F	Cerebral blood flow is likely to be reduced by >10% and even this may be poorly tolerated in an elderly patient.
	D – T	Pauses of >2 seconds should be viewed with caution as they carry an adverse prognosis for sudden death.
	E – F	Frequently seen in apparently normal people, but if their frequency is >10/minute they are associated with a poor prognosis in patients recovering from a myocardial infarction – there is an increased incidence of sudden death in such patients.
8.	A – T	Fixed-rate pacing at a rate slower than the tachycardia acts by rendering the circuit refractory; however, it is the least effective method of pacing for tachycardia.
	B – F	This method saturates the re-entrant circuit and is effective in atrial flutter and junctional arrhythmias. It may accelerate ventricular tachycardia or convert it to fibrillation.
	C – T	But it is a technique best left to experts as it requires specialist equipment to administer very precisely timed premature stimuli.
	D – F	Pacing at a rate faster than the sinus rate may reduce the tendency for recurrence once the arrhythmia has been terminated.
	E – F	Junctional tachycardias terminated by either; atrial arrhythmias are best terminated by atrial pacing.

9.
- A – T Some patients spontaneously vomit and this action terminates a junctional tachycardia. Ipecac. can be given to patients in whom vomiting is known to be effective.
- B – T It is unnecessary for the patient to actually immerse the head in water. This manoeuvre is highly effective in children.
- C – F This technique is not advisable as it is uncomfortable for the patient, is ineffective, and seldom works if other methods have failed.
- D – F The patient should be supine, carotid bruits should not be present and massage should be rotary or longitudinal.
- E – T Terminating about 50% of junctional arrhythmias. The patient should blow a sphygmomanometer to about 40-60 mm mercury and hold this for 15 seconds. The arrhythmia usually terminates during the relaxation after this.

10.
- A – F Supraventricular tachycardia is regular and slight variation in rhythm occurs with ventricular tachycardia.
- B – T However, the rapid rate in supraventricular tachycardia means the P wave and the T wave are often superimposed making it difficult to see. Occasionally, the P waves may be seen in ventricular tachycardia, but unlike supraventricular tachycardia, they will have no relationship to the ventricular complex unless a 'capture' beat occurs.
- C – T The P wave will only be seen with slower rates of ventricular tachycardia and will have a normal sinus rate of 60-100.
- D – F Vagal stimulation will only slow the ventricular rate in supraventricular tachycardia and has no effect in ventricular tachycardia.
- E – F Cannon waves are more likely to occur in supraventricular tachycardia with atrio-ventricular block, e.g. from digitalis; they are rare in ventricular tachycardia but may occur if an occasional atrial contraction coincides with the ventricular contraction.

11.
- A – F Atrial fibrillation is caused by enhanced automaticity. Atrio-ventricular re-entry is responsible for the paroxysmal supraventricular tachycardia.
- B – F Bundle of Kent insertion into the right ventricle (type B WPW) produces predominantly negative ECG in the chest leads.

C – F   WPW syndrome is always associated with a delta wave:
- type A – positive delta wave V1–V6
- type B – biphasic or negative delta wave V1–V3
- type C – positive delta wave V1–V4\: negative delta wave V5–V6

D – F   The bundle of Kent inserts into the normal myocardium and as a result ventricular activation initiates relatively slowly, thus accounting for the slurred upstroke or delta wave.

E – T   Digoxin enhances atrio-ventricular conduction in the accessory bundle and so increases the ventricular rate. Disopyramide is the treatment of choice since it slows conduction in both the accessory bundle and the normal A-V nodal pathway.

12.

A – F   Although verapamil may slow the ventricular response in atrial flutter/fibrillation it is unlikely to restore sinus rhythm.

B – T   Quinidine, like other class IA anti-arrhythmic drugs, is effective in both supraventricular and ventricular tachy-arrhythmia.

C – F   Although bretylium tosylate may be effective in aborting an acute attack of ventricular tachycardia, its long-term use is limited by side-effects such as postural hypotension. Its main use is for resistant ventricular tachycardia which has failed to respond to lignocaine and other conventional anti-arrhythmics.

D – T   Cardioversion is a very effective treatment of acute atrial flutter, often with a very small shock (25–50 joules).

E – F   There are two kinds of ventricular tachycardia in which verapamil may be very effective:
- (a) Gallavardin's benign repetitive ventricular tachycardia in the young.
- (b) Ventricular tachycardia associated with Prinzmetal's variant angina.

13. A – F   Hypothyroidism causes sinus bradycardia and heart failure but not atrial fibrillation: hyperthyroidism frequently leads to atrial fibrillation and should always be considered, especially in the absence of other evidence of heart disease.

B – T   Digoxin is contraindicated in atrial fibrillation with WPW syndrome because it may accelerate conduction in the accessory bundle and so increase ventricular response and precipitate heart failure and even ventricular fibrillation.

C – F   Anticoagulation may reduce the incidence of embolic stroke in AF irrespective of a rheumatic origin.

D – F   Cardioversion is only indicated if it is known that the AF is of recent origin, otherwise it may lead to systemic emboli; if in doubt, always use digoxin first (except in WPW syndrome).

E – T   Pericarditis is often associated with atrial arrhythmias like AF probably because of the proximity of the sino-atrial node to the pericardium.

CARDIAC SURGERY

14. A – F   Both these mechanical valves have a low incidence of mechanical failure and are reliable and long-lasting.

B – T   Most valves have a high incidence of thromboembolism if not anticoagulated – and many whether warfarinised or not, but in general all valves other than the tissue valves should receive lifelong anticoagulation.

C – F   Tissue degeneration is likely to occur from 7 years after implantation: destruction is rapid once it has presented and replacement should be carried out as a matter of urgency.

D – F   Prosthetic endocarditits is not related to the valve position and is more common in patients whose valve was replaced for bacterial endocarditis than for rheumatic or ischaemic disease.

E – T   Haemolysis may occur even in a mechanical valve is functioning normally, so the presence of haemolysis should alert the clinician to the possibility of a paraprosthetic leak.

15. A - F Even with currently used immunosuppressives, rejection occurs at least once in >90% recipients. Early signs of rejection include the development of third and fourth heart sounds and diminution of QRS voltages on the ECG.

B - T A pulmonary vascular resistance of >8 Wood units is a contraindication to transplant unless it is combined with a lung transplant, because this would rapidly cause right heart failure in the donor heart.

C - T Azathioprine and corticosteroids, the former at the highest level compatible with an adequate white cell and platelet count; the latter at the lowest dose necessary to prevent rejection.

D - T Nearly all patients sustain at least one infective episode. The majority are bacterial infections of the lung and usually correspond to high levels of immunosuppression and are commonest in the first 3 months after surgery.

E - F Accelerated atherosclerosis in the donor heart is a serious cause of late morbidity and mortality and may be reduced by low lipid diet, exercise and antiplatelet therapy.

CARDIOMYOPATHY

16. A - F Valve lesions are rare at necropsy. The myocardium bears the brunt of the disease, but the pericardium is commonly involved.

B - F Although ventricular arrhythmias may occur, the commonest presentation is with complete heart block, and sarcoid heart disease should be suspected in any young patient who suddenly develops complete heart block.

C - F Left ventricular aneurysm often develops as a result of the disease itself[4] and therefore should not be regarded as a contraindication to the use of steriods.

D - T The lesions tend to be patchy so that a negative biopsy does not exclude the diagnosis. Biopsy of skin, gland, bronchus, lung or a Kveim test are all helpful diagnostic tests.

E - F The echocardiogram may show dyskinesis, mitral valve dysfunction, septal thickening and bright echoes from the ventricular septum and left ventricular free wall consistent with fibrogranulomatous infiltration.

17. A – F PCM may present in the last few months of pregnancy as well as the first few months afterwards.
B – F It usually occurs in the third or subsequent pregnancy; it may occur in a first pregnancy if the patient is having twins.
C – T
D – F excessive salt intake has been found to be relevant only in African women, especially Nigerians.
E – T PCM may be caused by an acute auto-immune myocarditis, and on this basis immuno-suppressive treatment with prednisolone ± azathioprine has been found to be beneficial both symptomatically and on objective assessment by endomyocardial biopsy.

CARDIOTOXICITY

18. A – T Acute toxicity develops within a few days and is often transient: chronic cardiotoxicity occurs up to 28 weeks after starting treatment.
B – T The acute changes are mainly benign arrhythmias and are usually benign though an occasional death can occur as a result of myocardial infarction. Chronic cardiotoxicity causes the development of a degenerative cardiomyopathy and carries a high mortality.
C – T A cumulative dose of doxorubicin exceeding 500 mg/m^2 is more likely to lead to toxic effects.
D – F Although this ratio was initially thought to be a good indicator of toxicity, further studies have shown many false-positive results. The best non-invasive test is measurement of the left ventricular ejection fraction by radionuclide angiography: the best invasive test is subendocardial biopsy.
E – T The peak blood level of doxorubicin seems to be the most important factor determining cardiotoxicity; this is lower with continuous i.v. infusion than with intermittent i.v. boluses.

CLINICAL EXAMINATION

19.
- A – F   The mitral first sound, due to left ventricular systole, precedes the tricuspid sound because the right ventricle contracts just after the left ventricle.
- B – F   Inspiration widens the split between the mitral and tricuspid sounds by increasing the venous return to the right side of the heart, thereby delaying tricuspid valve opening.
- C – F   The first sound is louder if the P-R interval is short.
- D – F   The first heart sound may be louder in mitral stenosis but it does not split. The presence of an opening snap occuring shortly after the second heart sound in severe mitral stenosis may simulate splitting of the *second* heart sound.
- E – T   Aortic stenosis may cause slowing of the process of left ventricular contraction and so lead to softening of the first heart sound.

20.
- A – F   The third heart sound represents rapid filling of the left ventricle in early diastole.
- B – F   As the fourth sound is caused by atrial systole at the end of diastole, it will disappear in atrial fibrillation.
- C – F   A gallop rhythm is not uncommon in patients up to the age of 30 years, without indicating the presence of cardiac disease.
- D – T   A fourth sound is due to altered compliance of the left ventricle and is often heard in any condition causing an increase in end-diastolic pressure e.g. HOCM, aortic stenosis, hypertension. Its clinical significance is that it indicates left ventricular strain.
- E – T   May occur normally in young healthy adults and is thought to be due to sudden limitation of filling of the left ventricle. In older patients it is always abnormal and usually indicates failure of one or other ventricle.

21.
- A – F   Normally the aortic valve closes first and the later closure of the pulmonary valve is the cause of a splitting of the second sound.
- B – T   And the pulmonary component of the second sound is very faint.

C – **F**	The second sound will be fixed and split. The lack of splitting of the second sound may suggest Fallot's tetralogy, severe stenosis of the pulmonary or aortic valves, pulmonary atresia, a large VSD or hypertension.
D – **T**	The continuous systolic and diastolic murmur, heard at the left sternal edge, frequently obscures the second heart sound.
E – **T**	In transposition, the aortic second sound is both loud and palpable at the upper sternum, being generated from the anteriorly placed aorta – the pulmonary second sound is often inaudible due to its usual softness and its posterior placement.

22.
A – **T**	Febrile states such as typhoid cause intense vasodilation and a dicrotic pulse, even in the presence of a normal aortic valve.
B – **T**	This type of pulse is found in mitral regurgitation and ventricular septal defect, due to 'ventricular runoff'.
C – **F**	Although associated with aortic regurgitation, this abnormality may also be found in conditions of arteriovenous fistula, either natural or man-made, and in severe anaemia and thyrotoxicosis.
D – **F**	The paradoxical pulse, which is a rise in pulse pressure on *expiration*, is a feature of pericardial tamponade or acute, severe asthma.
E – **F**	Pulsus alternans is found with varying cardiac outputs in heart failure. Pulsus bisferiens is the abnormal notched pulse that represents a mixed aortic valve problem.

CONGENITAL HEART DISEASE

23.
A – **T**	70% of ventricular septal defects are small, and about 60% of these close during childhood; most of the rest become so small as to be clinically insignificant, and spontaneous closure in adult life is not uncommon. Only 20% of ventricular septal defects require surgical closure, usually within the first 2 years of life.
B – **F**	Although the majority of atrial septal defects remain asymptomatic, spontaneous closure is exceptional.

C – F If the ductus is small and the pulmonary artery pressure is normal asymptomatic survival into adult life is possible. However, chronic volume overloading of the left ventricle may lead to left ventricular failure in the child, and there is always the risk of infective endocarditis.

D – F 60% of infants with coarctation of the aorta have associated congenital cardiac defects, like ventricular septal defect, patent ductus arteriosus, congenital mitral valve abnormalities and bicuspid aortic valve.

E – F 90% of untreated patients with Fallot's tetralogy die before they reach 25 years. The average age of death is 5 years. Operative mortality is <5% and 75% of the survivors may live >30 years post-operatively.

24. A – F The pulmonary artery pressure is normal in coarctation; it is the systemic pressure which is increased (and reduced distal to the coarctation – hence the reduced or absent femoral pulses).

B – F A ventricular septal defect increases the oxygen saturation of the blood in the right ventricle: increased oxygen saturation in the right atrium is due to an atrial septal defect.

C – T Left-to-right shunting of blood from the aorta to the pulmonary artery increases the oxygen saturation. Right atrial and right ventricular oxygen saturation remain normal.

D – F The oxygen saturation in the left ventricle is reduced due to the right-to-left shunting; the right ventricular oxygen saturation may also be reduced due to return of de-oxygenated blood to the heart.

E – F The right and left ventricular pressure are often equal in Eisenmenger's syndrome allowing free flow either way across the septal defect. Closure of a ventricular septal defect in these circumstances is contraindicated and may be fatal because of the consequent increase in pressure in the right ventricle leading to right ventricular failure and death.

25. A – T The commonest symptoms are headache (due to hypertension), intermittent claudication or 'tired' legs on exertion (due to poor peripheral blood supply) or breathlessness (due to left ventricular failure).

B – F Associated lesions are common including bicuspid aortic valve, patent ductus arteriosus, ventricular septal defect and mitral valve abnormalities.

C – T Rib notching develops from the age of 6 years, and is caused by enlargement of the intercostal arteries acting as collaterals to divert blood from the subclavian arteries to the descending aorta below the coarctation (see Figure).

D – T Cerebral haemorrhage occurs due either to the hypertension or to a ruptured berry aneurysm which occurs commonly in coarctation.

E – F There is a spontaneous abortion rate of 25% in coarctation. There is only a minimal increase in maternal mortality, though occasionally dissection of the aorta may occur.

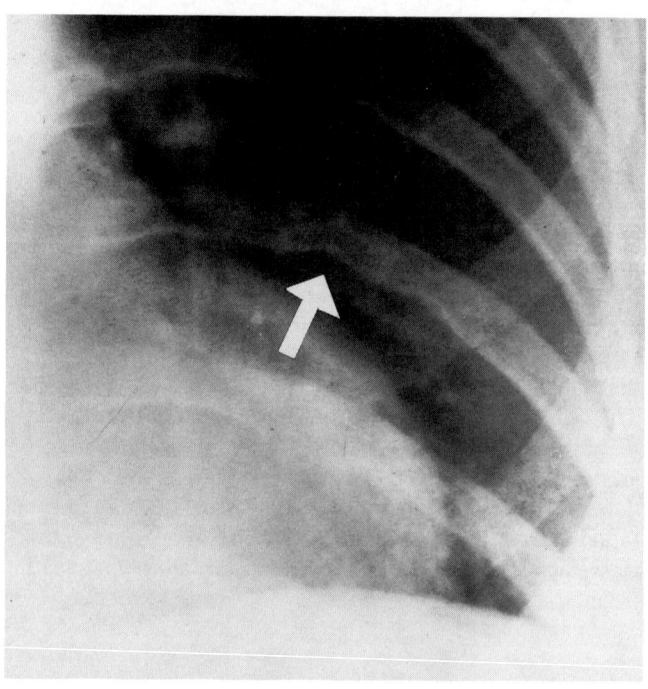

Chest X-ray showing rib notching in coarctation of aorta

MCQs in CARDIOLOGY

26.
- A – T Especially those premature babies who have the 'respiratory distress' syndrome.
- B – F PDA is the commonest congenital cardiac lesion associated with rubella infection in pregnancy.
- C – F PDA is usually asymptomatic and tends to be picked up for the first time at a school medical examination.
- D – T Eisenmenger's syndrome occurs in 5% of patients with PDA. It develops when severe pulmonary hypertension occurs leading to a reversal of flow through the ductus; in this condition the toes may become clubbed and cyanosed while the fingers remain unaffected.
- E – F PDA is pre-term infants is best treated by infusion of indomethacin which inhibits endogenous prostaglandins; prostaglandin infusion is used to keep the ductus open in conditions such as pulmonary oedema, so offloading the pulmonary circulation.

27.
- A – F A right-sided aortic arch is present in only 25%. Other associated congenital abnormalities include aortic incompetence and atrial septal defect.
- B – F Unlike transposition of the great vessels, cyanosis takes 3 to 6 months to develop in Fallot's tetralogy.
- C – F The 'a' wave is absent in Fallot's tetralogy: it is in isolated pulmonary stenosis that there is a giant 'a' wave and not when the pulmonary stenosis is a part of Fallot's tetralogy.
- D – F Total correction early in life is associated with a high mortality. The best treatment is a Blalock shunt initially followed by total correction when the child is 5-10 years old.
- E – T Squatting improves breathlessness by:
  (a) increasing systemic vascular resistance thereby reducing right to left shunting.
  (b) impeding the venous return to the heart from the constricted veins in the legs so reducing cardiac work.

28.
- A – F The incidence is higher than this at about 8 per thousand live births.
- B – F An isolated VSD is more common, affecting about 2 in every 1000 live births.
- C – F Spontaneous closure occurs in only 30–50% of patients.

D – T   This is the commonest cause of 'hyperkinetic' pulmonary hypertension, which will be evidenced by a chest X-ray showing pulmonary plethora and an enlarged pulmonary artery.

E – F   Less than 10% of patients with VSD also have a patent duct.

CORONARY SPASM

29.
A – F   There is a variable heart rate response. Inferior ischaemia is associated with a slight bradycardia whereas anterior ischaemia causes a tachycardia.

B – F   The LVEDP rises uniformly as the ischaemia persists, although systemic BP initially falls then rises in response to the continued pain.

C – F   Narrowings of 25–30% is frequently seen in such patients. It is believed that coronary artery spasm only rarely occurs in normal coronary arteries.

D – F   The aetiology is more complex and it is not known what is the cause. Active influences include endogenous vasoconstrictors and endothelial damage causing loss of endothelium-dependent vasodilator substances. These factors may influence the activation of vascular smooth muscle.

E – F   There is evidence that myocardial oxygen demand does not change, but 'supply' is reduced: ST segment elevation occurs in about 35% of patients during chest pain and ergometrine induces spasm in 15–20% of patients.

DRIVING LICENCE AND HEART DISEASE

30.
A – T   If it shows a conduction defect, evidence of ischaemia or ventricular enlargement.

B – F   As long as he has no side-effects from the medication, but if he is receiving anticoagulants he may not hold such a licence.

C – T   If the cardiothoracic ratio is >55% or more, a licence cannot be held; and neither can one be held if there is any evidence of cardiomyopathy.

D – T Whatever the other rhythm, whether sustained or paroxysmal.
E – T The above criteria (A–D) apply equally to patients who have had valve repair or replacement, single or multiple.

31.
A – F The licence should be suspended for 6 months after the first attack but may be restored if the patient remains free of recurrences.
B – T Sustained or recurrent atrial fibrillation is a bar to such a licence as there is increased incidence of stroke and peripheral embolism.
C – F If paroxysmal SVT occurs without dizziness or angina patients may hold a licence after cardiological review. Ventricular tachycardia is a bar to such a licence.
D – F Casual BP reading of 200/110 are a bar, but treated patients without postural hypotension or syncope may hold a vocational licence.
E – T Although normal driving is permitted in the presence of a pacemaker if regularly checked, a vocational licence cannot be held except in exceptional situations reviewed by an Honorary Medical Advisory Panel.

32.
A – T If there is >2 mm ST segment depression during a Bruce protocol when patient is *off* medication for 48 hours before the test.
B – T If there are persistent and typical Q waves lasting >40 ms and a height of at least a third of the succeeding R wave.
C – F If the exercise test is normal (<2 mm ST depression) after maximal exercise and a coronary angiogram shows single vessel disease involving a vessel other than the LAD. However, the granting of a licence in these circumstances depends on annual review and a normal maximal exercise test.
D – F Unless he has had one documented myocardial infarction as well, in which case a licence cannot be held.
E – T If the cardiothoracic ratio is >55% on a chest X-ray, the patient is barred from holding such a licence.

ECG

33.
- A – T Left axis deviation is said to occur when the cardiac axis is between −30 and −90 degrees. If the axis is between −90 and 180 degrees, extreme left axis deviation is present.
- B – T A secundum ASD typically causes a right axis shift on the ECG because of the right ventricular hypertrophy resulting from left-to-right shunting of blood.
- C – F The ostium primum ASD is associated with left axis deviation because of mitral valve involvement and the associated mitral incompetence leading to left ventricular hypertrophy.
- D – F Left axis deviation represents block in the anterior hemibundle; posterior hemi-block is shown as right axis deviation
- E – F Severe pulmonary stenosis may result in deviation of the axis to the right due to marked right ventricular hypertrophy.

34.
- A – T The prolongation is caused by both increased heart rate and increased catecholamine production on exertion.
- B – T And it can be corrected for heart rate (QTc) by dividing the measured interval by the square root of the cycle length.
- C – F The Lange–Nielson hereditary syndrome is recessively inherited and is associated with nerve deafness. The Romano–Ward syndrome is dominantly inherited.
- D – T Because of a tendency to develop ventricular tachycardia on emotion or exercise. This results in syncope and sometimes death.
- E – F As the cause is thought be to an imbalance between the sympathetic innervation on the right and left sides of the heart, full β-blockade may be effective in controlling symptoms.

35.
- A – T This is probably due to the increase in sympathetic tone produced by exercise.
- B – T The QT interval is dependent on the cycle length, and is calculated from the formula:
(measured QT interval)/(sq. root of the R–R interval)

C – F   The Romano–Ward syndrome is not associated with deafness; it is the Jerwell–Lange–Nielsen syndrome in which a prolonged QT interval is associated with congenital nerve deafness.

D – F   β-Blockers in full dose is the treatment of choice in ventricular tachycardia – characteristically 'torsade de pointes' – occurring with the prolonged QT syndrome. Isoprenaline infusion is indicated if torsade de pointes is associated with complete heart block.

E – F   It is aggravated by hypokalaemia and hypocalcaemia, and it is therefore important to look for and correct any electrolyte disturbance of this type in ventricular tachycardia associated with a prolonged QT.

FIBRINOLYSIS

36.
A – (a) iii   Recruiting 11,712 patients and mortality at 21 days.
B – (a) ii   Recruiting 1,741 patients and assessing the 21-day mortality.
C – (a) iv   Recruiting 17,187 patients and mortality given for 5 weeks.
D – (c) ii   Recruiting 1,004 patients; mortality at 30 days.
E – (b) i   5,011 patients and 28-day mortality figures.

37.
A – F   After TPA it does enhance the action of the drug and reduce rethrombosis but after the non fibrin-specific agents (streptokinase and APSAC), which themselves produce a hypocoagulble state, it is not essential.

B – T   And because of this, anticoagulants are less effective in arterial vessels than anti-platelet agents in preventing thrombosis.

C – F   The high rates of rethrombosis after fibrinolytic therapy are not reduced by the co-administration of heparin, which itself augments the platelet activation of lytic therapy.

D – T   The high-molecular weight heparins bind to platelets, causing activation and subsequent aggregation, thrombosis and thrombocytopenia.

E – F   Heparin activated antithrombin III blocks the action of thrombin in the blood but cannot inhibit fibrin formed on platelet surfaces.

38.
- A – F Compared TPA 100 mg/3 h to placebo in 5,011 patients with a history suggestive of MI within 5 hours of onset of main symptoms (ECG changes were not mandatory).
- B – T All patients had a heparin bolus at the time of administration of TPA and then an infusion of heparin for 24 hours. Aspirin was not given.
- C – T The 1 month mortality was reduced by 26%, from 9.8% to 7.2%.
- D – F Benefit with TPA was confined to patients who had ECG evidence of myocardial infarction.
- E – F Incidence of stroke was similar in both groups of patients, although haemorrhagic stroke was more common in the TPA group.

39.
- A – b Streptokinase immediately combines with plasminogen to form a fibrin binding chemical that converts plasminogen to plasmin.
- B – c APSAC (or Eminase) is a plasminogen-streptokinase activation complex which is activated by de-acylation which occurs after it is fibrin bound.
- C – a It is a direct activator of plasminogen.
- D – e This binds strongly to fibrin and acts as a cofactor in the activation of plasminogen.
- E – d A precursor of urokinase and converted to this before it can act.

HEART BLOCK

40.
- A – F The q wave is absent in the chest leads with left bundle branch block.
- B – F Left bundle branch block increases the risk of sudden death, especially if it is of recent origin.
- C – T If the left bundle branch block is confined to the left anterior fascicle.
- D – T If the left bundle branch block affects the posterior fascicle only.
- E – F Right bundle branch block is associated with septal defects, especially atrial septal defect. The only type of congenital heart disease in which left bundle branch block is frequent is idiopathic hypertrophic subaortic stenosis.

41.
- A − F There is no warning before the loss of consciousness and this helps differentiate it from epilepsy.
- B − T A tonic-clonic seizure may result from the cerebral hypoxia caused by asystole.
- C − T The collapse is associated with pallor due to arrested circulation but the recovery is often heralded by a profound flushing as the circulation returns and this is a characteristic feature noted by witnesses.
- D − T And the lack of a post-ictal phase helps to differentiate a Stokes–Adams attack from an epileptic seizure.
- E − F The episode of loss of consciousness is usually very transient and recovery is rapid.

HYPERLIPIDAEMIA

42.
- A − F Nicotinic acid acts by inhibiting the secretion of lipoproteins from the liver: cholestryramine binds bile acids in the bowel.
- B − T
- C − F Fibrates are less effective than nicotinic acid in reducing the cholesterol level but more effective in controlling hypertriglyceridaemia.
- D − F Gemfibrozil *potentiates* the action of warfarin.
- E − T

HYPERTENSION

43.
- A − F It occurs more frequently in women (70%) and has a peak incidence in the third and fourth decades. A history of hypertension in pregnancy is common in these women.
- B − F Conn's syndrome is most frequently picked up by detecting asymptomatic hypertension on routine examination. The hypertension is rarely severe and almost never malignant.
- C − F 80% of random blood samples will show hypokalaemia, and salt loading will unmask hypokalaemia in virtually all patients with Conn's syndrome.

D – T Patients with hyperaldosteronism due to adrenal hyperplasia remain under the control of the renin–angiotensin system and tilting into the erect position will therefore result in an increase in plasma aldosterone level – adenoma patients have no such response.

E – T The other 25% of patients will stay hypertensive, either because of pre-existing essential hypertension or from renal damage caused by prolonged secondary hypertension.

44.
A – F PPH is more frequent in women (2.5:1), probably because of hormonal influences. It can occur as a result of taking the contraceptive pill.

B – T The aetiology of PPH is unknown. Among the theories are recurrent pulmonary emboli from occult systemic venous thrombosis, vasculitis due to collagen disease, giant cell arteritis (Takayasu's disease), congenital defects in the pulmonary arterial wall and drug sensitivity reactions (penicillin, sulphonamides, chloramphenicol).

C – T Raynaud's disease occurs in 10-30% of patients with PPH.

D – F The commonest manifestations are a loud second heart sound (98%), cardiomegaly on X-ray (95%) and the ECG abnormalities of RV and RA hypertrophy (95%). The commonest symptom is breathlessness (75%), exertional dizziness (30%) and angina (8%)[10].

E – F Results are variable but successes have been reported with hydralazine, phentolamine, diazoxide and nifedipine; also intermittent i.v. prostacyclin may be of value. Probably the most useful treatment of all is long-term anticoagulation.

INFECTIVE ENDOCARDITIS

45.
A – F 50% of cases involve valves that were previously not known to be abnormal.

B – F Although *Streptococcus viridans* is responsible for about 75% of infections in the non-geriatric medical patients, this falls to 50% with an increase in *Streptococcus faecalis* and *Staphylococcus epidermidis*, and Gram-negative organisms from the bowel in elderly patients.

C – T   Multiple infection should be suspected if the initial response is followed by a relapse and a different organism is found in the blood culture.
D – T   Two antibiotics should be used for a synergistic effect and to reduce the development of resistant organisms. Benzyl penicillin combined with gentamicin is the usual starting combination unless staphylococcal infection is suspected, when flucloxacillin should be used.
E – T   6 weeks treatment should be the general rule and in the absence of complications, patients should usually have been afebrile for 14 days before treatment is discontinued. Straightforward *Streptococcus viridans* infections can usually be treated with 14 days intravenous penicillin and gentamicin, then a further 2 weeks of oral amoxycillin. *Streptococcus faecalis* should always be treated for 6 weeks with parenteral penicillin and gentamicin.

46. A   goes with (c)
B   goes with (a)
C   goes with (e)
D   goes with (a)
E   goes with (b)

Dental patients who should be referred to hospital as they are at special risk of endocarditis are those who have prosthetic valves and require a general anaesthetic, those with previous proven attacks of endocarditis and those who require a general anaesthetic and are allergic to penicillin. Cover for obstetric and gynaecological procedures and gastroenterological procedures only requires prophylaxis if patients have prosthetic valves.

47. A – T   Autopsy shows Libman–Sacks endocarditis in up to 40% of patients with SLE, though the clinical incidence is much less as the condition is often clinically silent.
B – T   The lesions usually affect the underside of the mitral valve. Aortic valve involvement can occur but is rare. The tricuspid and pulmonary valves are virtually never affected.

C – F   Although the typical lesions in both types of endocarditis are fibro-fibrinous verrucose vegetations, there may also be focal necrosis and mononuclear cell infiltration in Libman–Sacks valves.

D – F   Mitral regurgitation, and rarely aortic regurgitation, may occur when the valve lesion has fibrosed; actual stenosis of the mitral valve has never been reported.

E – F   Libman–Sacks endocarditis does predispose to infective endocarditis, especially if the patient with SLE is immunosuppressed by treatment with steroids.

48. A – F   Atrial septal defect is virtually never involved in infective endocarditis; it is common, however, in ventricular septal defect and patent ductus arteriosus prior to ligation, and may also occur in aortic coarctation.

B – F   A positive blood culture is found in abut 80%: a negative result should always raise the possibility of an unusual organism like coxiella (Q fever), brucella, aspergillus and candida.

C – F   Malignancy may cause marantic endocarditis which is not infective but likely to be due to tumour emboli.

D – F   *Streptococcus viridans* is still the most common infecting organism (about 50%); *Staphylococcus aureus* and *S. epidermidis* account for about 25% of cases.

E – T

MITRAL VALVE PROLAPSE

49. A – F   A floppy mitral valve is thought to be present in about 4% of the normal population.

B – T   Due to progressive stretching of the leaflets and weakening caused by deposition of acid mucopolysaccharides in the zona spongiosa.

C – T   And the impulse is thought to be caused by an increase in the tension of the chordae which occurs in the middle of systole.

D – T   The click occurs after the carotid upstroke of the pulse which helps differentiate it from a similar but earlier sound in aortic stenosis.

E – F The murmurs of MVP and HOCM are both accentuated after amyl nitrite – and HOCM does not have a midsystolic click and therefore may be differentiated from MVP.

50.
- A – F Mitral valve prolapse is found in about 5% of the normal population.
- B – F It does produce a 3rd sound but this is a systolic sound and resembles an ejection click.
- C – T Although frequently benign, mitral valve prolapse can lead to chest pain, cardiac arrhythmias, systemic emboli and even sudden death.
- D – F The condition is due to a myxomatous type of degeneration in the mitral valve and may also involve the aortic, tricuspid and pulmonary valves, as well as the myocardium itself.
- E – T

MYOCARDIAL INFARCTION

51.
- A – F Atenolol was compared to placebo; aspirin was a limb in the ISIS 2 trial with streptokinase.
- B – F Atenolol was initially given intravenously followed by an oral dose and mortality at 7 days was reduced by 15% compared to placebo.
- C – F Patients were included if they were within 12 hours of onset of symptoms: mean time to inclusion was 5 hours.
- D – F The incidence of VF and cardiac arrest was not reduced in the β-blocked group: 2.4% of treated patients had a non-fatal cardiac arrest compared to 2.5% on placebo.
- E – T 7-day mortality reduced by 15%, from 4.5% to 3.9% and this reduction was predominantly a reduction in ventricular rupture.

52.
- A – T 1.5 megaUnits SK infused over 1 hour and/or 160 mg aspirin per day for 1 month (or identical placebos in >17,000 patients presenting within 24 hours of an acute myocardial infarction.
- B – F Patients were recruited up to 24 hours after onset of their major symptoms.

C – F   Aspirin alone reduced mortality by 25% at 5 weeks from 12% to 9.2%.
D – T   Mortality reduction on combined therapy of 42%; from 13.2% to 8%.
E – F   Treatment was equally effective in the 20% of trial patients over the age of 70 years, and this improved mortality was maintained at up to 15 months after infarction.

53.
A – F   It used to be thought of merely as a reciprocal electrical eveclnt reflecting the extent of the ST elevation in opposite leads but now is believed to be a sign of ischaemia in other areas.
B – F   These patients have greater enzyme rises and more in-hospital complications that patients without this phenomenon.
C – F   There is no convincing evidence that reciprocal change does identify disease in arteries remote from the site of the infarction.
D – T   Although there may not be remote coronary artery disease, the ECG abnormalities may reflect a critical reduction in coronary flow in remote areas in patients at higher than usual risk of complications.
E – T   The area of reciprocal change is often the area where ST depression will occur on later exercise testing. Such patients may have significant coronary disease in this territory away from that of the infarction.

54.
A – F   Typical pericardial pain occurs in about 30% of patients, a rub is detected in up to 20%, but a clinically significant pericardial effusion is uncommon.
B – F   An effusion, of itself, does not appear to increase the mortality: however, as its occurrence seems to be related to larger infarcts, anterior infarcts and left ventricular failure, it would appear to be a marker for those patients at higher risk of death.
C – F   Although infrequently requiring drainage, an effusion may persist for 6 months after the infarction in a third of patients.

D – F There is up to 50 ml fluid in the normal pericardial cavity and this may be misdiagnosed as an effusion. Pericardial fat, a coronary fistula and a pericardial tumour may also be indistinguishable from an effusion.
E – T The fluid is thought to be the result of the oedema and inflammation that follows infarction and indicates the healing process is active.

55.
A – F 50% of patients dying after an inferior myocardial infarction are shown to have infarction of the right ventricle, and as much as 25% of the ventricular wall may be involved.
B – F Although this may be a manifestation of right ventricular infarction, it is neither sensitive nor specific. Even ST elevation in right precordial leads, although sensitive (>80%) has a specificity of between 40 and 90% so is unreliable.
C – F Severe RV dysfunction occurs in 10–20% of patients with RV infarction and has the characteristics of a right atrial pressure of >10 mm or a RA:Wedge pressure ratio of >0.8.
D – T It is fluids, rather than diuretics, that are required for the low output state that accompanies RV infarction. Always consider this possibility in a patient with inferior myocardial infarction followed by cardiogenic shock and be prepared to measure the left and right atrial pressures.
E – F The typical findings of hypotension, oliguria, raised jugular venous pressure with Kussmaul's sign and clear lung fields differentiates it from pure LV failure.

56.
A – T The cholesterol plaque ruptures, platelets are deposited, the coagulation system is initiated and red blood cells and fibrin are deposited.
B – F Red blood cell accumulation in the plaque without prior fissuring is not important as it is often found in controls. Plaque fissuring is usually the initiating event.
C – F 20–50% of patients with non-Q wave infarction are shown to have total coronary artery occlusion.
D – T Studies have shown that prolonged infusions of TPA may result in progressive increase in arterial lumen and decrease in stenosis, although in most cases a significant (>70%) stenosis of the occluded coronary artery remains.

E – T   It has been shown that it is the exposure of the type I collagen fibres deep in the arterial media which stimulates platelet aggregation and thrombus formation. This is fixed deep in the artery wall and is likely to occlude the lumen.

57.
A – F   Initially this was thought to be so, but their antiarrhythmic properties are minimal and other mechanisms are thought to be responsible.
B – T   The Norwegian study of timolol versus placebo[11] showed a 16.8% vs 10.4% reduction in mortality at a mean time of 17 months post-infarction. This was the first convincing and adequately controlled trial of β-blockers in myocardial infarction.
C – F   The BHAT study[12], compared propranolol to placebo after acute infarction and showed a reduction in mortality from 9.5% to 7% at a mean of 24 months.
D – T   Atenolol appears to prevent early death by reducing incidence of ventricular rupture, rather than preventing later death, as shown in the ISIS 1 trial[1].
E – T   Probably correct, but as there is no convincing evidence of benefit after 2 years, which is the longest time reported so far in any of the accepted clinical trials.

58.
A – T   In 60% of cases, associated with atheroma of the anterior descending artery and full thickness anterior myocardial infarction.
B – F   Only 20% of VSDs are in the posterior part of the septum and thus involve the mitral valve by infarction and rupture of the papillary muscles.
C – T   40% of patients who survive the acute phase of septal rupture develop aneurysmal dilatation of the remainder of the infarcted septum and ventricle.
D – F   66% occur within 3 days of infarction and the rest within 7 days of onset. 1–3% of myocardial infarctions are complicated by VSD and they account for 1–5% of deaths at the peri-infarct period.
E – F   25% are fatal within 24 hours of rupture and 50% are dead within 1 week. Less than 30% survive 2 weeks and only 20% are alive at 30 days. Without surgery, long-term survival is rare and early surgery is indicated.

59.
- A – F Autopsy studies have shown no consistent distinction between Q and non-Q wave infarction though in general Q wave infarction tends to be more extensive.
- B – F Non-Q wave infarction occurs more frequently in an older population. This is likely to be due to the increase in collateral circulation in the elderly leading to a more restricted infarction.
- C – F Although the short-term prognosis is better in the non-Q wave infarction, the long-term prognosis is the same.
- D – T Non-Q wave infarction comprises only 20–25% of myocardial infarction encountered in hospital practice.
- E – T A randomised controlled trial in 576 patients[13] reduced both re-infarction rate and mortality and the incidence of post-infarction angina with the use of diltiazem in non-Q wave infarction.

60.
- A – F QRS changes may be found in patients who are later shown histologically to have had a subendocardial infarction and so should not be relied upon in the clinical diagnosis.
- B – T Early transmural infarction is often found in patients thought to have had a subendocarial infarction and subendocardial infarction is considered by many to be an intermediate state between crescendo angina and transmural myocardial infarction.
- C – T Coronary vascular resistance rises with the high intramural tension in the subendocardium during systole. This virtually restricts perfusion of the subendocardium to diastole, and renders this zone vulnerable to ischaemic damage.
- D – T Aortic stenosis is related to this type of infarction because of a combination of reduced coronary artery perfusion and increased left ventricular diastolic pressure, as a result of left ventricular hypertrophy, both of which jeopardise the perfusion of the subendocardial zone.
- E – T Cardiac massage can maintain effective cerebral circulation but coronary circulation is reduced to as little as 15% of the carotid circulation. This type of infarct should be considered after successful resuscitation.

61. A – F   There is rarely a past history of angina.
B – F   Most of the patients are smokers.
C – T
D – F   Coronary spasm can be demonstrated in only a minority of the patients: other possible causes include coronary emboli from intramural thrombosis, small artery disease not visible on coronary arteriography and polycythaemia.
E – F   The exercise test is usually negative after the infarction.

MYOCARDITIS

62. A – T   Features suggestive of this include a 4-fold rise in antibody titre in paired sera and a type specific IgM with a titre of >1/32.
B – F   5% of patients suffering from a viral illness have cardiac involvement and histological evidence of viral myocarditis is present in 2–5% of unselected autopsies and 17–21% of patients with unexpected cardiac death.
C – T   In males, the young and the pregnant, presenting as a subacute illness after a viral infection.
D – F   Although the ECG is commonly abnormal, the changes are non-specific ST and T wave changes; arrhythmias and conduction disturbances may be the only sign of cardiac involvement.
E – F   Steroids and immunosuppressives given in the early stages of the illness may actually increase cardiac damage, and most patients recover completely without such treatment.

63. A – F   The P–R interval is *shortened* in approximately 50% of cases of Duchenne's muscular dystrophy, indicating *accelerated* conduction, possibly due to an accessory conducting bundle.
B – F   Atrial standstill is the distinctive cardiac complication of Landouzy–Déjèrine muscular dystrophy.
C – T   The myocardium is rarely involved enough to produce any clinical manifestations. On the other hand, the His–Purkinje system is affected in 80% of patients with myotonia dystrophica causing conduction defects.
D – F   Thomsen's disease is benign and the prognosis is good. The heart is very rarely affected.

E – F Hypertrophic cardiomyopathy occurs in 20% of patients with Friedreich's ataxia. As the septum is rarely involved in the hypertrophy – unlike the usual genetic type of hypertrophic obstructive cardiomyopathy – serious ventricular arrhythmias do not occur.

PERICARDITIS

64. A – F This only applies now to developing countries. In developed nations, most cases are of unknown aetiology but most likely due to earlier undiagnosed viral pericarditis (the exception is in young children where TB still accounts for the majority of cases).

B – F A prominent 'x' descent alone indicates cardiac tamponade. Both 'x' and 'y' descent are present and increased in pericardial constriction (see Figure).

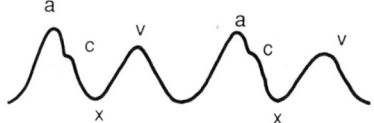

Normal jugular venous pulse

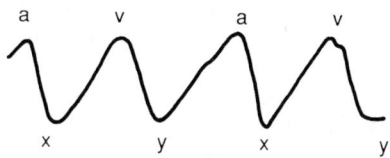

Jugular venous pulse in constrictive pericarditis showing prominent 'x' and 'y' descents

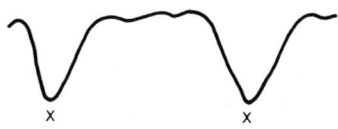

Jugular venous pulse in cardiac tamponade showing prominent 'x' descent but no 'y' descent

C – F Constrictive pericarditis is not associated with marked inspiratory swings in right ventricular filling pressure so pulsus paradoxus is usually absent.
D – F Left ventricular systolic function is normal in both restrictive cardiomyopathy and pericardial constriction.
E – T Complete resection of the pericardium is the best treatment with up to 85% 5-year survival. Diuretics are only of short-term benefit.

65.
A – T The heart size may be reduced if the pericarditis is constrictive; otherwise the heart size is normal.
B – F A paradoxical pulse indicates tamponade.
C – T
D – T Bronchial breathing may be heard at the left lung base if the pericarditis is accompanied by a large pericardial effusion compressing the left lower lobe (Ewart's sign).
E – F Kussmaul's sign is a *rise* in the jugular venous pressure in inspiration with a more prominent 'x' descent.

PHYSIOLOGY

66.
A – T ANF is produced mainly in the left atrial appendage in healthy individuals but ventricular secretion may occur in heart failure.
B – F ANF secretion is increased by an *increased* intake of Na and falls if Na intake is reduced – it helps to maintain a constant blood volume.
C – F ANF inhibits renin secretion and also attenuates the effects of pressor infusion of angiotensin II.
D – T The increase of ANF in heart failure is stimulated by the raised filling pressure in the ventricles as well as the Na retention.
E – F Effective diuretic treatment will *reduce* circulating blood levels of ANF.

RESUSCITATION

67. A – F Sometimes fine ventriclar fibrillation can simulate asystole, therefore it is always worth trying defibrillation with 200 joules (twice) then 360 joules before adrenaline 1 mg is given.

B – F DC shocks of 200 joules should be tried twice, then, if unsuccessful, a further shock of 360 joules should be given; if still unsuccessful, 1 mg i.v. adrenaline and a further DC shock of 360 joules given before 100 mg lignocaine is administered if the ventricular fibrillation persists, followed by further attempts at defibrillation.

C – F CPR may be interrupted but for no more than 10 seconds at a time, except for DC shock.

D – F CPR should be continued for 2 minutes after each drug before concluding that it has not been effective and a further agent administered.

E – T If an intravenous line cannot be obtained, medication should be given in double dosage through the endotracheal tube where absorption of the drug can occur through the tracheo-bronchial mucosa.

68. A – F It is better to nurse with the patient's head slightly elevated to prevent oedema gravitating towards the brain. Fluid retention should be vigorously treated with diuretics.

B – T Cerebral recovery is impeded by high or high normal blood sugars, which regulate the metabolism of the brain. It is necessary to aim to keep the patient's blood sugar at the lower end of the normal range, with insulin if necessary.

C – T It is thought beneficial to reduce the pCO_2 to 4 kPa (30 mmHg) for 36 hours in an effort to enhance recovery – the low levels of CO_2 are thought to improve the metabolic function of the brain.

D – F They should not be taken off a ventilator unless their cardiac rhythm is stable, they are free of pulmonary oedema and their blood gases are satisfactory.

E – T You should always be wary of a fall in heart rate and blood pressure as these may be the only signs of drug intoxication causing myocardial depression.

RHEUMATIC HEART DISEASE

69. A – T Aortic stenosis leads to an increase in left ventricular end-diastolic pressure, which is responsible for the exaggeration of the P wave (often inverted 'normally' in lead V1 of the ECG).

B – F The calcified aortic valve is above and anterior to the oblique fissure on the lateral chest X-ray.

C – F M mode echo is not reliable. Doppler gives a better idea of the degree of stenosis but the best method of assessment is direct measurement of the gradient across the aortic valve at catheterisation.

D – F The onset of symptoms is the time for surgery: the average survival is only 2–3 years with angina/syncope and only 18 months once cardiac failure has occurred.

E – F The commonest associations are with coarctation of the aorta (Turner's syndrome) or with coarctation and a patent ductus arteriosus as well.

70. A – F It may co-exist with an atrial septal defect in the inherited Lutembacher's syndrome, which may be confused with rheumatic mitral stenosis and a patent foramen ovale.

B – F The usual infecting organism is of the Group A streptococcal family (usually type 12) and the antigen–antibody reaction damages the valve.

C – F The catheter used for angiocardiography may cause parts of the myxoma to become detached and to embolise: the best test for diagnosis and differentiation is echocardiography.

D – T This is due to reduced cardiac output in patients with moderate or severe stenosis. On exertion, if the cardiac output is doubled, the gradient across the valve is quadrupled and increases the pulmonary capillary wedge pressure which restricts exertion. The presence of atrial fibrillation further reduces cardiac output.

E – T The enlargement of the left atrium will compress other structures such as the recurrent laryngeal nerve, resulting in hoarseness (Ortner's syndrome), compression of the oesophagus (dysphagia) and the left main bronchus (left lung collapse).

71.
- A – T The more stenosed the mitral valve, the softer is the first sound. A loud first sound is due to a 'still mobile' mitral valve being 'slammed' shut at the onset of ventricular systole.
- B – T The closer the opening snap is to the aortic second sound, the tighter the stenosis. This is because the left atrial pressure increases progressively with the severity of the mitral valve stenosis, and the higher the pressure, the earlier the mitral valve will open in diastole.
- C – F The more severe the stenosis, the longer the duration of diastolic flow and the murmur.
- D – F If mitral regurgitation co-exists and predominates, a third heart sound will often be audible.
- E – T This is thought to be due to oedematous bronchial mucosa which is prone to infection.

72.
- A – T If the jet is directed at the anterior wall of the left atrium.
- B – F Posterior chordal rupture causes the murmur to be heard best at the left sternal edge; anterior chordal rupture leads to a loud posterior murmur.
- C – F Mitral regurgitation is best seen by screening in the 30 degree right anterior oblique position.
- D – T The size of the left atrium is also related to the severity of the regurgitation. If the LA is greatly enlarged, it will 'absorb' some of the regurgitant pressure and so reduce the 'v' wave seen at catheterisation: this occurs in chronic, as opposed to acute, mitral regurgitation.
- E – T There is 60% survival at 5 years after diagnosis on medical treatment alone.

73.
- A – F Once symptoms occur and cardiomegaly is present on the chest X-ray prognosis is poor – the 3-year survival is only 65%.
- B – F Aortic regurgitation may result from an aneurysm of the sinus of Valsalva rupturing.
- C – T The Osler–Weber–Rendu syndrome may occasionally present with aortic regurgitation as well as cyanosis, bronchiectasis and secondary polycythaemia.

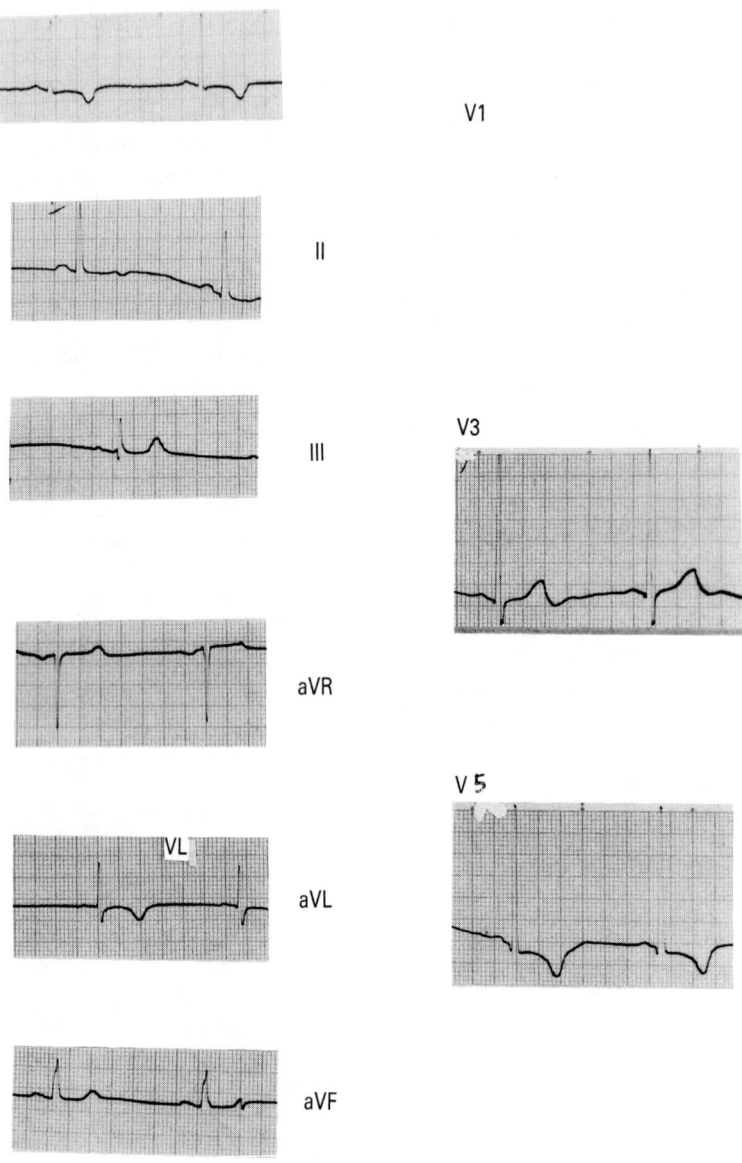

ECG in a patient with aortic regurgitation showing left ventricular strain manifesting as a tall R wave, ST depression and T inversion in V5

D - T The ECG may show left ventricular hypertrophy and a 'diastolic overload' pattern of prominent Q waves in the anterolateral leads. As the condition deteriorates, ST depression and T wave inversion occur (see Figure on left).
E - T If the cause of the aortic regurgitation is syphilitic. Calcification of the aortic valve in rheumatic or congenital aortic regurgitation is rare.

74. A - F Pericarditis occurs in about 30% of patients with rheumatoid arthritis, and many of these cases are associated with effusion – especially if rheumatoid nodules are also present.
B - F The mitral valve is the one most frequently affected in rheumatoid arthritis, with the aortic, tricuspid and pulmonary then involved in that order.
C - T Myocarditis is rarely a clinical problem, except when associated with amyloidosis secondary to the rheumatoid arthritis. Pericarditis and endocarditis are much more common than myocarditis as a manifestation of rheumatoid heart disease.
D - F Abnormal T waves are no more common in rheumatoid arthritis than in controls. The commonest ECG abnormality is first degree heart block; other ECG changes include left bundle branch block, atrial fibrillation and ectopic beats.
E - F The incidence of coronary disease is higher and is thought to be due to arteritis of the coronary arteries – the incidence in rheumatoid patients at autopsy is 20%.

75. A - F The *Graham Steel* murmur is an early diastolic murmur due to pulmonary regurgitation, and occurs in mitral stenosis. It is the *Austin Flint* murmur which occurs in aortic regurgitation and may be confused with the murmur of mitral stenosis: it is said to be due to diastolic oscillation of the anterior mitral valve leaflet at the junction of the regurgitant jet from the leaking aortic valve and the normal forward flow from the left atrium to the left ventricle.

B – F   It is *pulsus bisferiens* which indicates combined aortic stenosis and regurgitation, and is due to a percussion wave in systole followed by the reflected tidal wave of aortic regurgitation, producing a double-peaked wave. *Pulsus alternans* is alternating normal and poor pulse beats due to impaired left ventricular function.

C – T   *De Musset's sign* indicates a hyperdynamic circulation and is due to the large pulse pressure which occurs in aortic regurgitation.

D – T   *Duroziez sign* is a to-and-fro murmur occurring over the femoral artery. It is best elicited by compression of the femoral artry proximally to show the systolic murmur and distal compression to bring out the diastolic murmur.

E – F   Squatting raises the arterial pressure and therefore enhances the regurgitation and the diastolic murmur, while the Valsalva manoeuvre lowers the systolic pressure and thereby reduces the murmur.

76. A – T   The connective tissue defect in pseudoxanthoma elasticum produces floppy mitral valve leaflets: other features of the condition include peau d'orange skin, retinal angioid streaks and gastro-intestinal bleeding.

B – F   The mitral regurgitation in Hurler's syndrome is due to papillary muscle dysfunction: other features of the condition include coarse features, corneal clouding and mental retardation.

C – T   Marfan's syndrome also leads to connective tissue dysfunction producing a floppy valve, as well as elongation and rupture of the chordae tendinaea.

D – F   As well as dilatation of the mitral annulus in left ventricular failure, transient disturbance of papillary muscle function occurs.

E – F   This type of infiltration often involves the papillary muscle as well as the valve itself.

77. A – F   A bisferiens pulse will occur only if the aortic stenosis is associated with aortic incompetence. The usual pulse is slow-rising (plateau pulse).

B – F   The second sound will be reduced only if the stenosis is the valvular type; subvalvular aortic stenosis is associated with a normal second heart sound.

C – T
D – T Systemic emboli may occur in aortic stenosis, especially if the valve is heavily calcified: the brain and the retina are the commonest sites affected, so amaurosis fugax may be a presenting feature.
E – T

THERAPEUTICS

78. A – T It is metabolised in the liver and should be avoided in patients with liver cell impairment; captopril may be better as it does not undergo liver metabolism.
B – T And it is thought that these may be responsible for some of its toxic side-effects such as the rash, taste disturbance and proteinuria. Enalapril does not contain such groups and may therefore have fewer of these side-effects.
C – F Captopril may be of some benefit if patients with diabetic nephropathy have proteinuria; the reasons for this benefit are unknown.
D – F Enalapril may reduce the creatinine clearance in patients with congestive cardiac failure, but does not cause proteinuria; captopril, however, does lead to proteinuria in high doses and renal function should therefore be monitored carefully.
E – F Patients who have had a skin rash with captopril have been safely given enalapril.

79. A – T All β-blockers, whether cardioselective or not, can cause bronchospasm and are therefore contraindicated in asthmatic patients; calcium antagonists have no adverse effects on the bronchi and are therefore the treatment of choice in asthmatic patients with angina or hypertension.
B – F β-blockers may alter the ratio of high-density to low-density lipoproteins unfavourably, but the clinical implications of this change remain to be shown. The calcium channel blockers have no adverse effects on the blood lipids and are the treatment of choice if the patient has associated hyperlipidaemia.

C – F Verapamil and diltiazem are negatively inotropic and therefore contraindicated in cardiac failure, but nifedipine may be given as it does not affect myocardial contractility.

D – T And can also be used in combination with digitalis without toxicity. Verapamil and diltiazem, together with β-blockers, should not be used in patients with digitalis toxicity, and they should be used with extreme care in patients on digoxin, even if not toxic.

E – F Nifedipine should be avoided in cardiomyopathy, as well as aortic stenosis, as its vasodilator properties may increase the gradient across the obstruction. The other calcium antagonists and the β-blockers are not thought to do this.

80.

A – F Nitrates are contraindicated in HOCM for the treatment of angina because any measure which reduces left ventricular volume will aggravate symptoms in HOCM; nitrates produce peripheral venodilatation which results in less venous return and therefore a reduced left ventricular volume.

B – T Nitrates will reduce the diastolic filling of the already compromised heart by causing a reduction in the venous return from peripheral venodilatation, and this in turn results in a further fall in the cardiac output.

C – F Nitrates are safe in anterior infarction but may cause a critical reduction in the filling pressure of the right ventricle in inferior infarction; this may well result in clinical deterioration since the right ventricle depends on adequate filling pressure to maintain its function in an inferior infarction.

D – F Apart from amyl nitrite, there is no evidence that other nitrates cause a rise in intraoccular pressure, and they can therefore be used safely in glaucoma.

E – F Sudden withdrawal of nitrates may lead to a clinical syndrome similar to that previously seen at the weekends in munition-factory workers during the last war – severe headaches. Additionally, sudden death has occasionally occurred following sudden cessation of long-term nitrate therapy.

81. A – F   β-Blockers will result in reduced hepatic clearance of lignocaine and therefore increase the tendency to side-effects.

B – T   There is displacement of digoxin from protein bound sites in patients on quinidine, increased blood digoxin levels and therefore an increased tendency to digoxin toxicity.

C – F   The combination of more than one Class III agent increases the likelihood of a prolonged QT interval which in turn encourages 'torsades de pointes' ventricular tachycardia.

D – T   Each Class I drug will cause myocardial depression, both of conduction and of myocardial contractility and so thry should not normally be given together.

E – T   Diuretic-induced hypokalaemia may increase the risk of 'torsades de pointes' ventricular tachycardia, a possible side-effect of quinidine.

82. A – F   75% is absorbed rapidly and the rest is inactivated by organisms in the lower intestine prior to excretion.

B – F   Digoxin is lipid soluble and so crosses the blood-brain barrier, although this is thought to be of little clinical significance.

C – F   Digoxin does not bind to plasma proteins and has a half-life of about 36 hours.

D – F   Most of the circulating digoxin is excreted unchanged by the kidneys and so dosage restriction is necessary in patients with renal impairment.

E – T   The mechanism is unknown but hyperthyroidism, malabsorption syndromes, and drugs which interfere with absorption (such as cholestyramine, neomycin, rifampicin) may all be associated with low serum levels of digoxin.

83. A – F   This is a specific property of sotalol alone. All the β-blockers limit the production of tissue cyclic AMP and this gives them their anti-arrhythmic activity.

B – T   Stimulation of the central nervous system at night, when sympathetic tone is low, may result in poor sleep.

C – F   Atenolol < metoprolol < acebutolol in selectivity of cardiac activity, but all β-blockers cause some degree of bronchospasm, usually at higher doses, and all should be avoided or used with caution in patients with chronic obstructive lung disease or asthma.

D – F   Although high ISA may diminish the bronchospasm induced by β-blockade, it will also lessen the response of the airways to β-agonist inhalers – thus a cardioselective β-blocker would be the β-blocker of choice in patients with airway obstruction.

E – T   Labetalol also causes less bronchospasm, but the two major consequences are postural hypotension in high doses, and retrograde ejaculation in men due to relaxation of the bladder neck sphincter.

84. A – T   If the angina is due to coronary spasm the β-blockers may enhance that artery spasm, due to unopposed α-receptor activity; β-blockers should therefore be avoided in Prinzmetal's variant angina, the basis of which is severe coronary spasm.

B – T   When combined with nifedipine in the treatment of angina, or hypertension, they reduce the resultant tachycardia. However, they should only be combined with verapamil cautiously because of potential AV block.

C – F   β-blockers are less effective in the elderly and these patients are more prone to side-effects. These patients are better started on a mild diuretic.

D – F   Black patients respond better to vasodilators or the combined α- and β-blocker, labetalol. The young non-smoking white male pateint, with co-existent angina, is the best responder to β-blockers.

E – T   The ideal β-blocker would be long acting, cardioselective, effective in the standard dose, have a simple metabolic pathway (no liver metabolism, little protein binding, lipid insoluble and no active metabolites) and would be vasodilatory and either have ISA or be α-blocking. Atenolol meets nearly all those ideals, other than lack of intrinsic sympathomimetic activity.

85.
- A – F It has been found in clinical studies that propranolol has to be withdrawn in about 10% of patients and atenolol in 2%. Both can cause fatigue, cold extremities and worsening claudication, dreams and bronchospasm.
- B – F This side-effect is suprisingly rare if the correct contraindications (patients known to have suffered cardiac failure or to have poor cardiac function) are adhered to and proper patient selection occurs.
- C – T It has occasionally been found that when used as mono-therapy, hypertension may be aggravated. This is related to increased fluid retention in patients with low renin levels.
- D – T This is because of its high intrinsic sympathomimetic activity. Labetalol, because of its α-blocking action, also causes less bradycardia and fall in cardiac output.
- E – F Propranolol causes vivid dreams by this mechanism but dreams in patients on pindolol are thought to be caused by the insomnia resulting from the relatively high sympathetic tone at night which results from its high intrinsic sympathomimetic activity.

86.
- A – F The α-mediated rebound hypertension caused by clonidine withdrawal will be exacerbated by the presence of a β-blocker.
- B – T Reserpine acts by causing a depletion of catecholamines, so interfering with the sympathomimetic properties of the β-blocker, which may thus have reduced effects.
- C – T Cimetidine reduces hepatic blood flow so blood levels of propranolol, which is metabolised in the liver, will be increased. In patients on cimetidine it may be better to use β-blockers which are not metabolised in the liver, such as atenolol, sotalol and nadolol.
- D – T By combining a β-blocker with nifedipine, the reflex tachycardia induced by the fall in blood pressure is reduced by the β-blocker, thus enhancing the hypotensive effect of the nifedipine.
- E – T The fluid retention caused by the NSAIDs counteracts the hypotensive effects of the β-blocker.

87.
- **A – F** Although ouabain acts rapidly after intravenous therapy (within 1 hour), it is not absorbed orally, and if i.v. administration is effective, a switch to oral digoxin should subsequently be made.
- **B – F** The half-life of digitoxin is between 4 and 6 days, although its hepatic metabolism and gut excretion make it useful in patients with renal failure requiring glycosides.
- **C – T** It has similar actions and indications to digoxin but causes less gastro-intestinal upset – it is rarely used except when patients are intolerant of other glycosides.
- **D – F** Its maximum benefit is 2–3 hours after it has been given, and oral digoxin, which is rapidly absorbed, is likely to be just as effective – and cheaper.
- **E – F** Although digoxin is the preferred glycoside, it has a half-life of 1–2 days, which is why it can be administered as a once-daily treatment.

88.
- **A – F** Although dopamine must be given through a central vein because of its irritant effects on smaller veins, dobutamine may be given through a peripheral line.
- **B – F** Because it has no such effect, it is less likely to cause tachycardia than is dopamine.
- **C – F** The myocardial nerve terminals do not release noradrenaline in response to dobutamine, although dopamine does cause its release.
- **D – T** Dobutamine is the only inotrope that does not cause a severe tachycardia in usual doses.
- **E – T** Both dopamine and dobutamine cause peripheral vasodilatation which is a β-2 receptor mediated effect.

89.
- **A – T** This action is mediated through α-receptors in the vessel walls.
- **B – F** Intravenous isoprenaline causes a tachycardia due to stimulation of the β-1 receptors in the wall of the ventricle.
- **C – F** Noradrenaline is released from myocardial cells in response to stimulation by dopamine and not dobutamine.
- **D – T** This action is mediated through the stimulation of β-2 receptors in the walls of peripheral vessels.
- **E – T** However, although both β-1 and -2 receptors are affected, there is only a weak β-2 stimulating effect and most actions are β-1 mediated.

90.
- A – ii   This is cardiogenic shock and the vasodilator will lower the PCWP as the inotrope will improve the contractility of the heart.
- B – iii The vasodilator will reduce the PCWP and therefore cardiac work. A diuretic may be a useful adjunct.
- C – i   The inotrope will improve cardiac contractility. A vasodilator will lower the blood pressure and thus aggravate the situation.
- D – v   These parameters are normal and merely require observation.
- E – iv   Suggests fluid depletion and the need for volume expansion with saline or dextran.

91.
- A – T   Class IV agents, the calcium antagonists, act by increasing the duration of AV node refractoriness.
- B – F   Class III drugs (e.g. amiodarone and sotalol) actually increase the time taken for His-Purkinje fibres to undergo further depolarisation and so reduce the ventricular response.
- C – F   Class II agents, the β-blockers, primarily depress the sinus node and the AV node and have little direct action on the ventricular muscle through their β-1 receptors.
- D – F   Although Class Ia (e.g. procainamide and disopyramide) and Ic agents (e.g. flecainide, propafenone) do increase the refractory period, Class Ib agents (e.g. lignocaine and mexilitene) actually reduce the refractoriness of the His–Purkinje fibres.
- E – T   By inhibiting the fast inward sodium current, the upstroke of the action potential is inhibited and this delays the return of excitability.

92.
- A – T   Particularly with captopril, to reduce the first-dose hypotensive effect. Advise patient to take the first dose last thing at night or to stay in bed for some hours after taking the tablet.
- B – T   Especially in patients with heart failure and renal impairment, as significant potassium retention may occur, particularly in the first few days.

C – F This is not necessary unless there is a reason to suspect renal artery disease (e.g. young patient with severe hypertension resistant to usual therapy). ACE inhibitors may cause renal failure in patients with unexpected renal artery stenosis – especially if unilateral.

D – T Probably advisable for patients requiring ACE inhibitors for heart failure rather than hypertension because the former are more likely to be on diuretics and therefore prone to the adverse effects on renal function and serum potassium levels.

E – F But the dose of loop diuretics (e.g. frusemide and bumetanide) should be at least halved a day before the introduction of ACE inhibitors, to improve the vascular 'state' and so avoid postural hypotension. Any potassium-sparing diuretic should be withdrawn to prevent severe hyperkalaemia.

93.
A – F Nitrates are predominantly venous vasodilators and improve cardiac failure by reducing the venous return to the heart.

B – F Nitroprusside is equally effective for arterial and venous vasodilatation. It is rapidly active, has a short half-life and may quickly be titrated against response. It is also potentially toxic and should be infused for relatively short periods by a large central vein.

C – F Infusions of this sympathomimetic may cause hypokalaemia and increase the tendency towards arrhythmias.

D – F An infusion of nitrosprusside causes anaerobic metabolism and the subsequent build-up of lactate in the arteries causes a metabolic acidosis.

E – F Hydralazine is predominantly an arterial dilator and causes a reduction in blood pressure, a fall in afterload and a reflex tachycardia.

94.
A – F Nitroprusside is converted to thiocyanate and high levels of this inhibit the thyroid gland, causing a hypothyroid state.

B – T The conversion of the metabolites of the nitroprusside to cyanocobalamins enhances excretion and reduces toxic side-effects.

C – T It inhibits cytochrome oxidase in the liver, into which it freely diffuses, and causes hypoxic damage to hepatocytes.

D – F 90% of the free cyanide is erythrocyte bound and, due to cytochrome oxidase inhibition, interferes with aerobic metabolism.

E – F The metabolites of nitroprusside are renally excreted and have a long half-life of about 7 days.

95.
A – T Although disopyramide is primarily a Class I anti-arrhythmic drug, it also has some Class III action and prolongs the duration of the action potential.

B – F 50% is excreted through the kidneys.

C – T There is 90% bio-availability of disopyramide after an oral dose.

D – F In supraventricular tachycardia associated with the WPW syndrome, verapamil acts primarily in blocking antegrade conduction through the AV node, whereas disopyramide can effectively block conduction in both the AV node and the accessory bundle, so disopyramide is the more effective agent.

E – T Disopyramide may prolong the QT interval excessively in the presence of hypokalaemia and so precipitate 'torsade de pointes' ventricular tachycardia (the same problem has been documented with quinidine also).

96.
A – F Amiodarone blocks both α- and β-receptors in the heart in a non-competitive manner.

B – T

C – F The acute intravenous use of amiodarone does have negative inotropic effects due to its anti-adrenergic actions and the drug should therefore be used carefully if left ventricular failure is present: chronic oral treatment does not depress cardiac function.

D – T

E – F The plasma concentration of amiodarone is halved in 3-10 days, but its complete elimination can take 1-4 months.

MCQs FOR GENERAL PRACTITIONERS

97.
- **A – F** Although non-selective β-blockers do reduce the awareness of hypoglycaemia, selective agents are less likely to do so and may be given – β-blockers may increase the blood sugar levels by up to 1.5 mmol/litre and doses require adjustment accordingly.
- **B – F** Non-selective β-blockers without intrinsic sympathomimetic activity (e.g. propranolol, sotalol, nadolol) should be avoided but β-blockers with high ISA, e.g. pindolol, or cardioselective agents, may be given.
- **C – T** Agents with low hepatic clearance, such as atenolol, nadolol, sotalol and pindolol, can safely be used. If plasma protein levels are reduced, then β-blockers that are highly protein bound, such as propranolol or pindolol, should be avoided.
- **D – T** β-blockers with a reasonable indication may be continued throughout the perioperative period. If the indication is trivial, they should be stopped 48 hours before surgery, as they may result in excessive bradycardia, heart failure and other effects possibly enhanced by an interaction with anaesthetic agents.
- **E – T** Although severe asthma is an absolute contraindication, patients with mild bronchospasm or chronic airways obstruction may receive cardioselective agents with the co-prescription of β-2 stimulants.

98.
- **A – T** The lack of first-pass metabolism of the mononitrates means a more predictable response to therapy than the dinitrates, which undergo variable hepatic metabolism to mononitrate, which is the active component.
- **B – F** The constant, relatively high blood levels caused by wearing the patch are thought to be responsible for nitrate tolerance and reduced efficacy of the drug. A nitrate-free interval, often during the night, is now recommended.
- **C – T** Nitrates do reduce coronary spasm, but also cause dilatation of peripheral veins, reducing venous return and so limiting cardiac work – it is this effect which is most important in relieving angina.

D – T Their effect in reducing 'preload' benefits patients with cardiac failure by 'unloading' the circulation and so reducing cardiac work.

E – T The hypotension caused when nitrates are combined with both β-blockers and calcium antagonists may make the patient feel worse, even if the angina is well controlled.

99.
A – F There is no warning before the loss of consciousness and this helps differentiate it from epilepsy.

B – T A tonic-clonic seizure may result from the cerebral hypoxia caused by asystole.

C – T The collapse is associated with pallor due to arrested circulation but the recovery is often heralded by a profound flushing as the circulation returns and this is a characteristic feature noted by witnesses.

D – T And the lack of a post-ictal phase helps to differentiate a Stokes-Adams attack from an epileptic seizure.

E – F The episode of loss of consciousness is usually very transient and recovery is rapid.

100.
A-b Carditis incidence 50%
B-a Arthritis incidence 80%
C-c Chorea incidence 10%
D-d Erythema marginatum incidence 5%
E-e Chronic heart disease incidence 30%

Comment

A Acute rheumatic carditis results in an initial mortality of 1%. It is often asymptomatic but may present as congestive cardiac failure. The rheumatic process remains active in the heart for 3 to 4 months usually but may last up to 6 months in a severe case.

B The arthritis is a migratory large joint arthritis affecting, in order of frequency, ankle, knee, wrist, hip and shoulder. The pain is usually of sudden onset reaching a peak in 12 to 24 hours; swelling is minimal. The migratory process lasts 3 to 6 weeks, and any one joint is rarely affected for longer than a week.

C	Chorea usually occurs after a 'latent' period of 3 to 6 months after the initial streptococcal infection; the ESR and ASO titres may therefore be normal at the time of onset of the chorea. Girls are more commonly affected than boys and symptoms may last for about 6 months with occasional severe cases up to 1 year.
D	Erythema marginatum consists of bright pink macules with a raised serpiginous edge; the rash affects the limbs and the trunk.
E	If recurrence of rheumatic fever is prevented by long-term prophylactic antibiotic therapy 70% of patients who develop an acute rheumatic carditis will have normal hearts.

101.

A – F	Most atrial septal defects are not hereditary. There is a rare hereditary syndrome, however, the Holt–Oram syndrome, in which there is a combination of atrial septal defect and congenital skeletal abnormality of the forearm (tri-phalangeal thumbs).
B – F	It is delayed closure of the pulmonary valve which causes the fixed splitting of the second heart sound in atrial septal defect: this is the result of the overfilling of the right ventricle by the shunt leading to prolongation of right ventricular systole and delayed closure therefore of the pulmonary valve.
C – F	Congenital pulmonary and aortic stenosis may co-exist in William's syndrome (elfin face, hypercalcaemia, mesenteric artery stenosis and rubella syndrome); this condition is very rare and often remains asymptomatic.
D – F	Finger clubbing is not found in children under 3 months old, even if the child is severely cyanosed.
E – T	The diastolic murmur is due to stretching of the pulmonary valve associated with the pulmonary hypertension occuring in Eisenmenger's syndrome. Systolic murmurs are unusual because of the equality of pressure in the two ventricles.

102. A – F Digoxin is an inotropic drug, i.e. a drug which increases the force of myocardial contraction. A chronotropic drug is one which alters the heart rate e.g. adrenaline or other β-receptor agonists (positive chronotropism).

B – F The value of digoxin in treating heart failure with sinus rhythm remains controversial; it is always worth considering if the heart failure fails to respond to other standard treatment like diuretics, vasodilators, ACE inhibitors, etc.

C – T Carbenoxolone causes a fall in serum potassium level and may therefore enhance toxicity due to digoxin, especially in the elderly.

D – F Digoxin is dangerous in atrial fibrillation due to the Wolff–Parkinson–White syndrome because it *increases* conduction of the atrial impulses down the accessory bundle, thereby speeding up the ventricular response and the development of heart failure.

E – T Digoxin is excreted by the kidneys and renal impairment reduces excretion and raises the blood digoxin level with the attendant risk of digoxin toxicity, especially in the elderly whose renal function is likely to be impaired anyway.

103. A – T The calcium antagonists reduce myocardial contractility by depriving the myocardial cells of an adequate supply of calcium ions which are necessary for the contraction of the myocardium (as well as all other muscles).

B – T By relaxing the smooth muscles in the systemic arteries leading to dilatation of the arteries, a fall in the peripheral resistance and a reduction of blood pressure, which reduces the work of the heart. Nifedipine is the most potent vasodilator of the calcium antagonists.

C – F The calcium antagonists reduce the heart rate by slowing conduction in the atrioventricular node – they have no significant effect on the sino-atrial node.

D – T They may improve intermittent claudication or Raynaud's disease: this effect is mediated by the vasodilatation induced by these drugs as a result of relaxing the smooth muscle in the arterial wall.

E – F Verapamil, and to a less extent nicardipine and diltiazem, are contraindicated because they may aggravate the heart block in the atrioventricular node. Nifedipine, however, has no significant effect on A-V nodal conduction and so may be used safely in patients with heart block.

104.

A goes with (e)
B goes with (d)
C goes with (c)
D goes with (b)
E goes with (a)

H.I. Quincke (1842–1922) German physician from Frankfurt. Introduced lumbar puncture as a diagnostic test.
Sir Dominic Corrigan (1802–1880) Famous Dublin physician. Was President of the Irish College of Physicians.
A. De Musset (1810–1957) French poet who had George Sand as his mistress before she left him for Chopin.
L. Traube (1818–1876) German physician from Silesia. Also described pulsus bigeminus in 1872.
P.L. Duroziez (1826–1897) French physician from Paris. Contemporary with Charcot.

105.

A – F About two-thirds of patients present with pain but they have other presentations. In contrast, the vast majority of young patients with an infarction present because of pain.

B – F Only a small proportion of patients can be said to have a truly 'silent' infarct (2% in a recent study[5]). The mechanism is possibly a reduced sensitivity to pain in the older patients.

C – F Acute dyspnoea is the second most common presenting symptom of myocardial infarction in the elderly. The overwhelming dyspnoea may 'mask' the pain in the patient's perception and so present like a 'silent infarction'.

D – F Mortality rises with age but so does the difficulty in recognising the diagnosis. Accurate diagnosis is necessary before appropriate treatment is essential, so it is essential to consider the possibility of an atypical presentation in an older patient.

E – F The fibrinolytic trials have shown that the benefits of treatment continue at all ages treated and as the elderly have a worse prognosis in view of their age, they are likely to have more to gain from such therapy.

106. A – F The major benefit of controlling hypertension, whether severe (diastolic pressure >115) or mild (DBP 100–115) is the reduction in the incidence of stroke: heart failure and renal failure may also be prevented. There is no convincing evidence, however, from any of the acceptable clinical trials of a reduction in the incidence of myocardial infarction, either fatal or non-fatal.

B – F 95% of the patients will have essential hypertension, and many of these patients will have a family history of hypertension, which is a useful diagnostic help when considering the cause of hypertension.

C – T An IVP is indicated only if there is a past or present history of renal disease, if a renal artery bruit is heard or in patients whose hypertension proves very difficult to control.

D – F The incidence of phaeochromocytoma is very small, only 0.1% of the hypertensive population. Estimation of urinary catecholamines is indicated only if there are suggestive symptoms, like paroxysmal headache, sweating, palpitations etc.

E – T The IVP changes which suggest renovascular hypertension are a smaller kidney, delayed excretion and denser contrast on the ischaemic side.

107.
- A – F The main beneficial action of nitrate preparations in angina is through their venodilating effect; this results in pooling of blood in the limbs with less venous return to the heart (pre-load), resulting in less cardiac work.
- B – F This used to be thought the case before widespread use of coronary arteriography showed clearly that coronary artery dilatation can occur with nitrates in diseased arteries as well as in healthy coronary arteries.
- C – F Tolerance is only likely to occur with continuous use of transdermal nitrate preparations. Although it may occur with long-term use of oral nitrate, this is very rare.
- D – T The conversion of dinitrate to mononitrate on first passage through the liver suggests that it may be better to use isosorbide mononitrate for therapy in the first instance to ensure more consistent nitrate blood levels.
- E – F Trinitrate spray and sublingually are equally effective in treating angina. The advantage of prescribing a spray in preference to the sublingual preparation is the longer 'shelf' life.

108.
- A – T Thiazides may increase the blood cholesterol level; this has not been found with the loop diuretics. Whether this lipid-raising effect has any adverse long-term clinical effects has not yet been shown.
- B – F Extra potassium is necessary only if very large doses of loop diurectics are used; in these circumstances potassium replacement is better achieved with a potassium-sparing diuretic, like amiloride or spironolactone, than by giving extra potassium tablets.
- C – T The recent MRC trial of treatment of mild hypertension[6] showed a 30% incidence of impotence in young male hypertensive patients. There is no evidence that loop diuretics have a similar effect.
- D – F Thiazides act on the distal tubules; loop diuretics act on the ascending limb of the loop of Henle.
- E – T Elderly patients often become weak after a successful diuresis, due primarily to a depletion of the circulating blood volume. Occasionally, in more severe cases of diuretic-induced weakness, hypokalaemia is a contributory factor, especially if the patient's potassium intake in the diet is deficient, as may often be the case in elderly patients living alone.

109.
- A – T All the diuretics in common use act in this way: most act directly on the renal tubules, e.g. thiazides, loop diuretics, but others, like spironolactone, exert their effect primarily by blocking the sodium-retaining action of aldosterone leading to the same end result.
- B – T Loop diuretics like frusemide do act as mild venodilating agents which produce a beneficial pooling of blood in the extremities in patients with heart failure.
- C – F The fall in serum sodium levels produced by diuretics leads to depletion of the circulating blood volume which in turn stimulates an *increased* production of renin and angiotensin.
- D – T Thiazides are more effective than loop diuretics in lowering blood pressure because they can act directly on the peripheral blood vessels and produce dilatation with a fall in peripheral resistance – the important factor in long-term control of hypertension. Loop diuretics do not have this vasodilating effect.
- E – F Thiazides and loop diuretics can increase the serum uric acid level and sometimes precipitate clinical gout. Other diuretics, like chlorthalidone, triamterene, amiloride and spironolactone, have no hyperuricaemic effect.

110.

A – F No adequate trials have been performed of anti-coagulation after myocardial infarction, although the Dutch '60-plus' study[7] showed that the stopping of warfarin, previously given for acute myocardial infarction, resulted in a highter fatality rate than if warfarin was continued.

B – T ISIS 2[2] showed that aspirin used alone or in conjunction with streptokinase reduced mortality in a dose of 160 mg daily.

C – T The only study showing any benefit[8] was when it was combined with aspirin – and there was similar benefit from aspirin alone.

D – F Trials of mexilitene, disopyramide and aprendine failed to show a reduction in mortality, even though they do suppress arrhythmias. Also, they tend to be pro-arrhythmic and negatively inotropic, both of which may have adverse effects on mortality.

E – F The Anturane Reinfarction study[9] initially supported this conclusion but a large number of ineligible patients were entered then deleted from results. When reanalysed on an 'intention to treat' basis, there was no difference between the groups.

REFERENCES

1. Wilcox RG (For ASSET Study Group). Trial of tissue plasminogen activator for mortality reduction in acute myocardial infarction (ASSET). *Lancet*, 1988, **2**, 525-33
2. ISIS 1 Collaborative Group. *Lancet*, 1986, **2**, 57-66
3. ISIS 2 Collaborative Group. *Lancet*, 1988, **2**, 349-60
4. Fleming HA. *Br. Med. J.* (Editorial), 1986, **292**, 1095-6
5. Bayer AJ et al. *J. Am. Geriatr. Soc.*, 1986, **34**, 263-6
6. MRC working party. MRC trial of treatment of mild hypertension: principal results. *Br. Med. J.*, 1985, **291**, 79-104
7. Sixty Plus Reinfarction Group. *Lancet*, 1980, **2**, 989-94
8. Persantin-Aspirin Reinfarction Study Group. *Circulation*, 1980, **62**, 449-61
9. Anturane Reinfarction Trial Research Group. *N. Engl. J. Med.*, 1980, **302**, 250-6
10. Fuster V, Steele PM, Edwards WD et al. Primary pulmonary hypertension. Natural history and the importance of thrombosis. *Circulation*, 1984, **70**, 580
11. The Norwegian Multicentre Study Group. *N. Engl. J. Med.*, 1981, **304**, 801-7
12. Beta Blocker Heart Attack Research Study Group. *JAMA*, 1982, **247**, 1707-14
13. Gibson RS, Boden WE, Theroux P. Diltiazem and re-infarction in patients with non-Q wave myocardial infarction; results of a double-blind randomised multicentre trial. *N. Engl. J. Med.*, 1986, **315**, 423